Nursing Home *Ethics*

Everyday Issues
Affecting Residents with Dementia

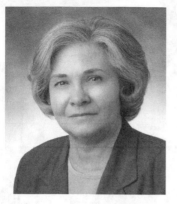

Bethel Ann Powers, RN, PhD, is an Associate Professor and Associate Director of the Center for Clinical Research on Aging at the University of Rochester School of Nursing in Rochester, New York. Dr. Powers received a BS degree in nursing from Alderson-Broaddus College in Philippi, West Virginia and an MS in nursing as well as MA and PhD degrees in anthropology from the University of Rochester. Her clinical work as a staff nurse and head nurse at Montefiore Hospital in New York City and as a nursing supervisor at The University of Rochester Medical Center has included care of older persons with terminal cancer, general medical and neurological problems, and rehabilitation needs. She joined the faculty at the University of Rochester School of Nursing in 1980. For the past 23 years, she has conducted clinical research focused on the culture of nursing homes, and more recently has focused on issues involving care of nursing home residents with dementia, through a variety of funded projects. She has received the Distinguished Nurse Researcher Award from The Foundation of the New York State Nurses Association (NYSNA) and the NYSNA Council on Nursing Research and an Excellence in Nursing Research Award from Epsilon Xi Chapter, Sigma Theta Tau International, Nursing Honor Society; and she is a Fellow of the Society for Applied Anthropology and The Gerontological Society of America.

Nursing Home *Ethics*

Everyday Issues
Affecting Residents with Dementia

Bethel Ann Powers, RN, PhD

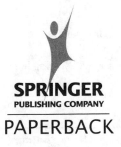

SPRINGER
PUBLISHING COMPANY

PAPERBACK

Springer Publishing Company, Inc.
11 West 42nd Street
New York, NY 10036

Acquisitions Editor: Helvi Gold
Production Editor: Janice Stangel
Cover design by Mimi Flow

06 07 08 09 / 5 4 3 2 1

New ISBN 0-8261-0270-0 © 2006 by Springer Publishing Company, Inc.

Library of Congress Cataloging-in-Publication Data

Powers, Bethel Ann, 1943-
        Nursing home ethics : everyday issues affecting residents with dementia /
Bethel Ann Powers.
                p. cm.
        Includes bibliographical references and index.
        ISBN 0-8261-1964-6
        1. Dementia—Patients—Care. 2. Nursing home care—Moral and ethical
aspects. I. Title.
RC524.P69 2003
362.2'3—dc21   2003050411

Printed in the United States of America by Bang Printing.

To those who pass through the mists of dementia,
May you know the warmth of love
And the comfort of the light of life within you,
For illness cannot claim your spirit.

And to those whose passage is complete,
May you walk forever in the light
With perfect understanding,
For the mists cannot pursue you.

This book is dedicated to persons with dementia;
to families and friends who share their journey;
and to the nursing home personnel who care for them.

Bethel Ann Powers
April, 2003

Contents

Foreword

Nursing homes are an essential part of the health care system, yet they have long been ignored and even demeaned. In *Nursing Home Ethics: Everyday Issues Affecting Residents With Dementia,* Bethel Ann Powers lays out in thoughtful and comprehensive ways the many ethical issues that arise in long term care. The first two chapters nicely review the conditions for which nursing home care becomes a necessity. By placing long term care in the context of individuals suffering from dementia and their family care providers, Dr. Powers helps the reader understand the emotional family context in which long term care takes place. These two chapters provide a wonderful introduction to the major focus of the book, the ethical stance that underlies long term care. Particularly useful in the section on ethical issues, in my opinion, is the practical nature of Dr. Powers' discussion. Rather than focusing on any single bioethics approach, she identifies common and uncommon events and uses them to develop an approach that is understandable, practical, and directly relevant to practicing in the long term care setting.

I can only hope that books like *Nursing Home Ethics* will bring long term care into the mainstream of the health care system. Dr. Powers reminds us that the provision of long term care is both necessary and rewarding and, as the number of individuals with dementia increases, long term care will be even more necessary whether it is carried out in nursing homes, assisted living facilities, or private homes. Dr. Powers' combination of practical advice, principled idealism, and prescriptive guidance makes *Nursing Home Ethics* a useful and necessary book.

Peter V. Rabins, M.D., MPH
Baltimore, MD

Introduction

The perspective advanced by this book is that living with and caring for persons with dementia in an institutional setting can be seen as an exercise in everyday ethics. Although primarily written for those who work in nursing homes and for educators and students in the field of gerontology, its content is presented in a way that can be appreciated by others as well. The writer invites this. In particular, the first two chapters on living with dementia and the nursing home experience may be of interest to a broader readership (such as laypersons or beginning level students and professionals). Chapter 3, on ethics in action, is more tailored to the needs of professionals. But, from this point on, families of persons with dementia might be interested in and consoled by descriptions of approaches that could be taken by a nursing home to understand residents' behavior and arrive at comfortable solutions. In addition, the practice cases in Chapter 4 are written intentionally at a general public reading level so that they may be used to meet in-service learning needs of certified nursing assistants and other nursing home personnel.

This book takes up where *The 36-Hour Day* (Mace & Rabins, 3rd ed., 1999) leaves off. *The 36-Hour Day*, although primarily written as a guide for laypersons and families caring for persons with dementia at home, is an invaluable resource to any individual whose personal interest, life circumstances, or professional commitment involves a desire to be as well-informed as possible in this area. These individuals include, for example, professional care-providers and educators who also may find its approaches to common issues and its understanding of the needs of both care-receivers and caregivers helpful. *Nursing Home Ethics* begins with the at-home experiences of persons with dementia that *The 36-Hour Day* explores in greater detail. However, it uses these experiences differently to appreciate how families try to sustain togetherness and to understand how they may come to the decision to pursue institutionalization. It then moves on to explore how approaches to previously encountered care issues (as told from the perspectives of residents, families, and staff members) become more complex in the nursing home environment, bringing persons new possibilities and challenges as they continue to struggle with the inevitability of disease progression.

This book also may serve as a companion to *Practical Dementia Care* (Rabins, Lyketsos, & Steele, 1999), another excellent reference guide for clinicians involved in caring for persons with dementia across the stages of their disease and across settings. Its holistic approach is developed around four perspectives: the disease perspective, dimensional characteristics of people with dementia, a behavioral approach, and a life story approach. *Nursing Home Ethics* focuses on a fifth perspective that involves careful consideration of the ethical implications of human relationships in everyday action within the specific context of nursing home culture. This perspective emphasizes the importance of understanding persons with dementia, their families, and nursing home staff members as unique individuals who may share common challenges but respond to them in different ways. To various extents, these responses are shaped by personal values, needs, and differences, as well as by the nature of institutional life.

In spirit, this book unites with others' efforts to draw attention to the importance, difficulty, and complexity of dealing with a major, devastating health care problem. Professionals in the field of dementia care differ in background, at times engaging different audiences on a variety of topics. However, they share a common motivation. That is, because they witness the suffering of persons affected by dementia, they naturally are concerned about public policy decisions that have an impact on the future of dementia care. Thus, they see an urgent need for persons in positions of power and authority (and their public supporters) to appreciate and "understand the skills involved in providing care for persons with dementia" (Rabins et al., 1999, p. 4). I join my colleagues in hoping that books like this will be useful to health care administrators, policy makers, and an informed public interested and willing to commit to improving care and quality of life for persons with dementia.

PROLOGUE

Different streams of experience have contributed to the writing of this book. Twenty-three years ago (1980), research on social support and social networks of elderly institutionalized people marked the beginning of my study of nursing home culture. At the time, I was interested in the abilities of "health-related facility" residents to manage their daily lives and sustain supportive relationships. In many instances, these were cognitively intact persons whose main reason for being in the nursing home was a lack of community-based options to forestall their admission. If the persons who taught me their "survival skills" then were here today, their places of residence, more likely, would be community-based in some sort of home care/assisted living type of arrangement. The nature of the nursing home population has been changing over the years in the direction of older, more acutely ill, physically frail, and cognitively impaired long-stay residents combined with a rapid in-and-out flow of short-term-stay residents who come for convalescence and rehabilitation or for palliative end-of-life care. And many more nursing homes are part of a "campus" offering multiple levels of care (i.e., home/day/respite care services, cottage/apartment independent living, select service options/assisted living, and a multiservice level nursing home: skilled care/rehabilitation/hospice). I think some of the participants in my network study would have been much happier living outside of the nursing home with some of these options. Conversely, I think that their lives probably would be more challenging in the midst of today's complex and needy nursing home population mix. And then I reflect on the idea that, in spite of all this change over time, there still are people in nursing homes who do not want to be and should not have to be there. Thus, lightly woven into this book is the assertion that the long-term care system, in which nursing homes play a vital role, still is out of balance. People at all socioeconomic levels should have better quality and more sustained opportunities for community-based care.

Few would disagree that it is good to support people's wishes to avoid having to live in a nursing home. But for persons with dementia and their families this represents a double-edged sword. Many persons with dementia have less cause for frustration and often function better in familiar surroundings. But, on the one hand, worries about their well-being may precipitate a nursing home admission because of others' discomfort about their safety. And, on the other hand, their health and safety may be placed at risk along with that of family caregivers when the latter press beyond the limits of their endurance in an effort to maintain the persons at home. Other persons with dementia may find the social pressures of familiar home surroundings confusing and threatening as their dementia progresses. Admission to a nursing home may relieve the pressure for such individuals. But the person with dementia is not in the best position to realize this and families may be unsure or divided in their opinions over when this transition from community to nursing home should take place. I have tried to capture the different kinds of experiences that underlie this dilemma, using quotes from taped interviews and field notes from my recent study of ethical issues affecting nursing home residents with dementia.

Nursing homes are challenging places in which to live and work. I was fortunate to serve on a nursing home ethics committee that committed itself to exploring the recurring everyday issues that make that so. The experience motivated the research project that produced the herein-described taxonomy of everyday ethical issues. The committee also became the reviewer panel that read and discussed the hypothetical case examples at the end of this book. When we began, there were few nursing home ethics committees to use as models. Our local counterparts were hospital ethics committees that did not mirror our circumstances and needs. Thus, over the years, the committee also has modeled much of what is described in the appendix as useful directions for the formation and function of such a group.

AUDIENCE

Persons who work in nursing homes are as diverse as the individuals in their care, not only in terms of appointment and job classification, but also in terms of education, experience, sensitivity, and temperament. Therefore, some issues discussed in this book that may be seen as commonplace and manageable by some staff members, may represent to others circumstances that are new and disturbing. Nursing home personnel vary considerably in their understanding of and comfort level in caring for residents with dementia. Mandated training programs for certified nursing assistants (CNAs), who provide the majority of hands-on care in nursing homes, devote little time to this topic. This means that understanding how to work effectively with these residents is mainly a matter of on-the-job training and in-service learning opportunities that will vary across nursing homes. Other persons with special learning needs may include lay volunteers, spiritual care providers, and board and committee members whose experiences and responsibilities external to the nursing home have not included an orientation to dementia care. Their personal satisfaction, continued service, and effectiveness may be limited by inability to recognize special needs of residents with dementia or discomfort with residents' affect or behaviors. Family members also may have difficulties in understanding issues surrounding the care of loved ones. Therefore, nursing home administrators, nurses, social workers, and service directors might want to share portions of this book with persons as a way of helping families understand the complexities and competing goods of nursing home life for individuals.

In fact, it could be empowering for families as well as comforting to know that they are not alone in this experience. Additionally, nursing homes may use the book to bring groups of individuals together in a meaningful exchange of thoughts and ideas about common issues and concerns.

Educators and students in the field of gerontology are important to our future as coparticipants in the development of service providers and policy makers in aging and long-term care. We need dedicated individuals whose lifework will be involved with finding solutions for specific problems encountered by elderly persons, improving existing care and service systems, challenging societal inequities, and developing innovative new approaches that promote and improve intergenerational harmony. This upcoming professional generation's understanding of issues related to dementia care is essential, especially as the number of persons affected by these diseases increases proportionally with the rising number of elderly in the general population. Therefore, this book's illumination of issues concerning residents with dementia, their families, and nursing home staff constitutes needed and highly appropriate subject matter for persons from various disciplines who are involved in this area of specialization.

BOOK FORMAT

Chapter 1 describes what living with dementia can be like, drawing on prenursing home memories of experiences provided by family members. However, it weaves these memories into an outline containing information that everyone ought to know about this condition: prevalence, multiple causes, onset and warning signs, and the reasons for and content of a skilled diagnostic evaluation with follow-up. It continues by laying out the issues of planning ahead, supporting persons with dementia in the community, and disease stages and symptoms leading to exploration of alternative residential care options. Overall, through systematic use of the words of persons who have lived through these experiences, it attempts to establish a tone that portrays the thoughts and emotions, the hopes and the fears that are part of this journey for families with persons they love.

Anthropologists use the personal down-to-earth writing style found in this chapter when they want to convey more than factual information. Thus, those who are new to this material will benefit from both the information and the insights provided. But readers who are familiar with the information should try to leave their minds open to the feelings expressed. For example, they might imagine themselves in the kinds of situations described or ask themselves if any of their own experiences (similar or dissimilar) have evoked corresponding kinds of feelings. And then they might consider whether identifying with others' feelings in these ways increases their appreciation of actual persons affected by dementia that they already know. No one can lead another person to this effort. Some come naturally; others refuse. But, from a human science perspective, regularly practicing such reflective techniques with the intent to become more thoughtfully attuned to the nature of an experience enhances sensitivity that can be helpful in building accepting, understanding, ongoing relationships with residents and family members.

Chapter 2 addresses the nursing home experience, mainly through the eyes of nursing home residents and their families. "Placement" is a term that is avoided here because it is denigrating to think of people as objects being "placed" somewhere. But family members struggle with this concept nonetheless, because nursing home admission most often is a decision that falls to them. Thus, this chapter tries to illustrate feelings about the transitions of persons with dementia to the status of "resident" and of family members to the role of "advocate." Most residents do not see this new place as their "home" because it is not familiar and often lacks recognizable homelike qualities. Characteristic features that constitute the cultural context of everyday issues are described in terms of how residents with dementia, in particular, are affected.

Some persons who work in nursing homes will derive new information and insights from this chapter. Others may view its contents with a sense of familiarity. However, what is described here is not being seen through their eyes. Therefore, it may benefit them to reflect on others' perceptions. In the human sciences, purposeful reflection requires the active participation of the reader with the written text. The text may remind readers of familiar experiences and their own responses and reactions to them. Thoughtful reflection on these experiences involves trying to view them from different perspectives, mentally reviewing and going over remembered details, and questioning their meaning. Questioning occurs not only in terms of how involved individuals were affected, but in terms of how experience teaches or raises concerns about how persons should be and act towards one another in different kinds of situations. In this manner, the text in Chapters 1 and 2 serves as a vehicle that moves sophisticated readers to higher levels of thought and deliberation over facts and issues that for others serve a more informative and sensitizing purpose. These chapters also set the stage for the specialized focus of Chapters 3 and 4.

Chapter 3 discusses the meaning of ethics in action as a practical approach to understanding everyday issues affecting nursing home residents with dementia. It addresses perceptions about the nature and intent of ethical deliberation as well as different analytic approaches that may be used. This time, contextual considerations that are offered address organizational features that affect ethical analysis of resident-focused cases (i.e., staff members' views about their work, organizational subcultures, and universal moral concerns). A framework to organize thinking about resident-focused cases is described. This taxonomy of everyday ethical issues shows ways to conceptualize the moral character-istics of ordinary concerns. (The figure of the taxonomy from the journal publication of my research is used with the permission of Lippin-cott, Williams & Wilkins.) Hypothetical cases illustrate each of the four domains, which are crosscut by dimensions of individual/social values and positive/negative rights. These cases are not so much for the pur-pose of analysis. They are exemplars whose purpose is to support discus-sion about the types of issues they represent and the kinds of questions that need to be asked when performing an analysis of a case. The compatibility of the taxonomy with Jonsen, Siegler, and Winslade's (1998) classic hospital-focused case analysis method (adapted to a nurs-ing home setting) also is discussed. The focus remains on persons with dementia, even though it is recognized that the taxonomy could work equally well for residents without this diagnosis.

Readers with a reflective grasp of resident-family experience, as encouraged in Chapters 1 and 2, may benefit the most from this chapter. However, each chapter can stand on its own. Here the reader is introduced to the idea that ethical deliberation is not cut and dry. Different analytic approaches are described and a particular way of thinking about how to draw on the best of these traditions is suggested. Thus, those seeking a rigid formula adhering to a single tradition will be disappointed (although they can consider reasoning that suggests why this may not be the best idea). But, through demonstration of how to use the taxonomy, they will find a structured method that can be followed. Learners new to the material should sample suggested readings that inform the discussion about the case examples. The maximum benefit for more experienced readers will be in going beyond the case examples to think about real situations within their own experiences and to apply suggested readings and others of their type to the different nuances of those cases.

Chapter 4 consists of twelve hypothetical cases. The topics go beyond previous examples, and the format is one of "dialogue" (questions and possible actions) and "commentary" (remarks in response to questions and possible actions). It is hoped that the conversation resists closure, since its purpose is to encourage ongoing dialogue around ethical issues in the care of nursing home residents, particularly those with a diagnosis of dementia.

The introduction to this chapter suggests a variety of ways in which this case material can be used—informally through individual reading and formally through group discussion. I believe that it is better for readers to consider the "dialogue" before reading the "commentary" because the idea is to encourage active, original thinking. The "commentary" should not be accepted passively. It represents the kind of response another might give. Readers may agree or disagree, but, in any event, they should be prepared to move on to new thoughts and ideas about the types of situations posed. That is, after all, the purpose of these exercises—to begin to demonstrate what an ethical case discussion could be like.

Note: *The study that generated many of the quotes appearing in this book was approved by an Institutional Review Board (IRB) responsible for overseeing and protecting the rights of human research subjects. Participants are not identified to maintain confidentiality and protect their privacy. Participation was voluntary and involved signed and witnessed consent forms containing information to help persons decide if they wished to be in the study, including their rights as research subjects, confidentiality of records, and dissemination of study results. The hypothetical cases are fictitious and do not represent actual persons or events. However, the commonly occurring situations and ethical issues that they depict are drawn from the true experiences of multiple nursing home residents, family, and staff members.*

Appendix—A question-answer format is used to discuss five topics: the why, where, what, who, and how of a nursing home ethics committee. Building on useful lessons learned by one committee, it reflects on ways to promote and energize committee activities. It is written as a conversation that must remain open because each nursing home's experience is unique.

ENDNOTE

The current volume is based on ethnographic research that sought to understand the experience of dementia, the culture of nursing homes, and how these phenomena interface in everyday life for residents, families, and staff members. An aim of this type of research is to present perspectives that are, at the same time, both common and ordinary as well as worthy of thoughtful contemplation. The author believes that the latter action is in itself an ethical activity. The narrative styles used are typical of the ways in which anthropologists apply their craft. On a personal note, however, the tone I have attempted to maintain throughout is intended to be one of respect for and fellowship with professional readers, one of the audiences for whom the book is written. Discussion of issues that persons who work in nursing homes encounter on a daily basis attests to the fact that theirs is not an easy path. I hope the narrative is at least validating, at best thought-provoking, and, ideally, of practical use. I further hope the book may prove useful to the extent that it may be shared with other persons, such as family members, who nurses or social workers identify as having various difficulties with situations they and their loved ones in nursing homes are encountering. And to educators and students, the other audience for whom the book is written, I hope that it is a good resource for those entering the field of gerontology who would seek to learn more about dementia and long-term care. There is such a desperate need for dedicated professionals in service to the growing elderly population—our parent generations, companions, and teachers. As God wills, we all will be old some day. Let us work to make each day better for growing older than the one before.

Bethel Ann Powers
April, 2003

Acknowledgments

I am grateful to the New York State Department of Health, Bureau of Long-Term Care, which funded the study that led me to write this book about ethical issues affecting nursing home residents with dementia. Many of the residents who participated in the study have since died. But the valuable lessons that they, their families, and nursing home staff members have taught me about what living with dementia and experiencing life in a nursing home are like are living testimonies of the courage, grace, and good humor of all these participants in the face of many challenges. I am deeply grateful to them for their wisdom, candor, and friendship. And also, to the ethics committee, which cannot be identified by name in order to respect the privacy of all, my heartfelt thanks.

Jeffrey Spike, Director of the Division of Medical Humanities at the University of Rochester Medical Center, is a valued colleague and mentor who has given graciously of his time in the course of the study and the preparation of manuscripts. His expertise as philosopher, ethicist, and ethics committee chair is deeply appreciated.

A number of colleagues and friends also contributed generously to this work by reading portions of the manuscript and giving constructive criticism. Mary Hauptmann, Paula Henry, Roberta Maruschock, Elaine Hiscock, Sharon Boyd, Jane Greenlaw, and Phoebe Thomas-Downing provided helpful advice from their professional and family perspectives on dementia and issues in long-term care. Many thanks also to University of Rochester School of Nursing colleagues in the Center for Clinical Research on Aging—Nancy Watson, Diane Mick, Hong Li, and Craig Sellers; and to Roger Kurlan, Professor of Neurology, University of Rochester School of Medicine and Dentistry, Alzheimer's Disease Center. I am grateful for the advice and support of Dean Patricia Chiverton and Bernadette Melnyk, Associate Dean for Research and Director of the Center for Nursing Scholarship and Evidence-Based Practice. And I also am indebted to friend and colleague Joel Savishinsky, Charles A.

Dana Professor in the Social Sciences, Department of Anthropology and the Gerontology Institute at Ithaca College.

Finally, thanks for editorial support to Judith Baggs, Marjorie Vandenberg, Theresa Kent, and Allison Calkins at the School of Nursing and to Helvi Gold and the editorial staff at Springer Publishing Company. Special thanks is given to my family. As always, I appreciate the love and support of my husband, Richard Powers, and my daughter and son-in-law, Rachel and Jeffrey Wilson, as well as the faith in me shown by my parents, Donald and Elizabeth Cornell.

Living With Dementia

OVERVIEW

This chapter examines the experience of living with dementia through the retrospective accounts of family members. First, their memories of onset and warning signs preface a discussion of considerations in diagnosing this condition. Second, a focus on interventions aimed at helping individuals compensate for some of the effects of cognitive impairment illustrates associated family dynamics and concerns. Third, stages and symptoms leading to exploration of alternative residential options precede examples of remembered difficulties of decisions associated with nursing home admission.

In the United States, an estimated 10% of adults aged 65 and older (and nearly half of those over 85) have Alzheimer's disease—the most common form of dementia (Alzheimer's Disease and Related Disorders Association [ADRDA], 2001a). Furthermore, although predictions about the number of cases in the absence of a cure vary widely (an increase from 4 million to between 8–14 million by mid-century), all projections consistently point to significant general escalation (ADRDA, 2001a; Evans et al., 1992; U.S. General Accounting Office, 1998). Even the authors of a recent report on the potential of advances in treatment that may delay onset and reduce overall prevalence of Alzheimer's disease reiterate the seriousness of rising disease trends: "None of our models predicts less than a threefold rise in the total number of persons with Alzheimer's disease between 2000 and 2050" (Sloane et al., 2002, p. 213). While Alzheimer's disease is the cause of about 70% of dementia cases, many other diseases account for the remaining 30%; for example, Lewy body disease and vascular dementias (Cullum & Rosenberg, 1998). Therefore, the number of persons suffering from dementia will be even greater than that predicted for Alzheimer's disease alone. Persons with dementia are not the only ones affected. When surveyed, 37 million

Americans knew someone who was so afflicted; and 19 million reported that these were family members (ADRDA, 2001a). Families, friends and neighbors generally are the first to notice and respond to the needs of elders whose independence and lifestyles are threatened by cognitive decline. Furthermore, this involvement often produces challenges and unanticipated changes in helper lifestyles and well-being.

"IT WAS SUCH AN UNEXPECTED THING."

Dementia is a broad classification denoting a cluster of clinical symptoms that can be caused by a number of specific diseases and conditions that interfere with the brain's ability to function at its usual level. This noticeable decline in previous ability is the feature that distinguishes dementia from preexisting conditions, such as mental retardation. However, the nature and speed of onset is unpredictable. (See Rabins, Lyketsos, & Steele, 1999, for categories of dementia and glossary of associated terms.)

> A daughter recalls: "It was such an unexpected thing to have happen to Mother. I was really surprised. To us it seemed sudden. [But I think] she knew something was wrong with her and she was worried about it."

People with early signs of dementia may sense that something is wrong but not communicate their concern to others. Some may suspect Alzheimer's disease (the most commonly known type of dementia), particularly those well familiar with the symptoms. Others may be unsure and wonder if memory lapses and/or difficulty in performing common, ordinary tasks are simply the signs of a slowing down that they associate with normal aging. Fear or lack of insight may cause people to minimize and deny problems. Also, it is not unusual for individuals to try to conceal evidence of problems they may be having. Those with good social skills are especially successful at preventing detection of memory loss and mental confusion or discovery of what they fear others may see as "mistakes." But the progressive nature of many types of dementia makes concealment more and more difficult over time. Sometimes those closest to the individual will be the most sensitive to changes in mood or behavior. However, closeness also may delay recognition or acceptance of early warning signs, as in the case of the companionable familiarity to be found in relationships that have weathered a lifetime of changes.

Wife: "It's hard to say exactly when [he showed signs of cognitive decline] because it was so gradual. I was with him all the time so it kind of crept up on me more slowly than it did for our daughter. She noticed before I did and asked, 'Don't you think Dad has failed quite a bit?' And I said, 'Oh well, but that's normal.' His memory just quietly left him. [His personality] didn't change much, but he just withdrew from things that he had enjoyed doing . . . just kind of a slow withdrawal."

Mild and gradual changes may not be apparent on routine medical examination. People who experience the following warning signs should be thoroughly examined by a medical specialist (neurologist or psychiatrist) or a comprehensive geriatric clinic team especially trained to evaluate memory problems:

1. Asking the same question or repeating the same story, word for word, over and over again.
"She was driving my father crazy asking the same questions over and over and over again."
2. Forgetting how to perform familiar activities (e.g., operating appliances, cooking, following written directions, telling time).
"First she told us there was something wrong with the clocks in her house. She got two or three new watches with great big numbers so she could read them better. She wanted a clock with great big numbers on it. And this was just an ongoing thing. She never said, 'I'm frightened.' She'd say, 'I've got to get another clock.' Now we realize how scared she must have been. Why is it people need to keep up pretenses? You know, 'You'll be okay, Mom. Sure, we'll get you another clock, and everything will be fine.' That was our hope."
3. Getting lost in familiar surroundings.
"She'd get confused coming out to the kitchen [or] she'd turn the wrong way to go to the bathroom."
4. Misplacing personal or household objects.
"He would hide things and then accuse me of taking them. And he was so inventive about where he hid things. I almost drove myself crazy looking and looking. Some things I never did find."
5. Accumulating and hoarding objects.
"I was not prepared for the mess my mother's house was in. I found package after package after package of things she had bought and never opened that had ended up in the basement."
6. Neglecting hygiene and personal appearance.
"It was hard to accept because Mom was a very meticulous person. There was not a hair out of line; and the clothes had to be right. When we were kids, too,

we always had to look sharp—clean, neat, and pressed. [When that changed] we knew something was going on."

7.   Having difficulty with/forgetting to take medications.

"She got very mad when I tried to do her pills. But it was obvious that she couldn't. We got a big weekly pill dispenser and put the pills in for each day—morning and night. But then we noticed one night that the pills for the next morning were gone. We suspect she may have taken her pills, gone back to bed, got up again, and taken the next day's pills."

8.   Having difficulty with driving.

"He [physician] said my mother shouldn't be driving. He said he had gotten a call from the police or the State or someone. Anyway, I guess she was getting lost. That was the first inkling [of a cause for concern]. Of course, she said he didn't know what he was talking about."

9.   Losing ability to write, read with understanding, handle money, pay bills, or balance a checkbook.

"She was dissatisfied and worried about things. And then she asked me if I would write her checks for her; and I saw what a mess her checkbook was in. We all have our pride and she didn't want to admit she was having trouble with it. So I would go up once or twice a week and see what mail she had and write checks for her bills. She would ask me to read some of the letters because she wouldn't understand what the communication was about."

10.   Losing ability to reason and to make informed decisions.

"He was spending money like it was going out of style, and then entering all these contests. But when he'd receive the books and the cassettes, he never opened them or anything. He'd just leave them in the box. He'd have mail all over the kitchen table, and I wasn't allowed to touch it because he said he knew where everything was. Then I knew something wasn't right. And I begged him, 'Please don't do it because you're not going to win anything.' Oh, and then he'd show me these letters that he'd get saying he was their number one candidate for the money. And I'd say, 'Honey, it isn't so.' But you couldn't convince him."

11.   Having increasing difficulty with following conversations and finding the correct words to convey information.

"She is able to see, and she can read words aloud, although she doesn't read everything exactly right. She's more interested in flipping through magazines for the pictures. And she'll react to some. Like she always loved little kids and she'll start to say something . . . like there was a picture of a little boy with his thumb in his mouth. But a lot of times the words don't come out right when she tries to verbalize. And she tried to say, 'Oh, look at what he's doing.' But she couldn't say that he was sucking his thumb. [Also, correct use of proper names and relationships causes difficulty.] I think she knows who I am [son], but she very rarely says my name."

12. Having increasing difficulty expressing abstract thoughts and feelings accompanied by changes in behavior (e.g., decreased responsiveness, increased irritability, suspiciousness of others, misinterpretation of what others say or do).

"A number of years ago, she very abruptly ditched all her old friends. None of them understood why, and the ones who are alive today still don't know why. None of us do. But now I'm very suspicious that this could have been the start [a warning sign]. I wonder if my mother could sense that something was going on and didn't know what. It's possible because she's very intelligent . . . very perceptive."

There are several good reasons to avoid delay in seeking competent professional evaluation of the above symptoms. First, these warning signs are not conclusive evidence of a dementing disease. There could be other underlying reasons for them that, once identified, will need to be addressed. Second, an early diagnosis of dementia enables institution of treatment in an attempt to slow the progression of the disease or to ease distressing symptoms (e.g., sleep disturbances, depression, agitation). Third, diagnosing dementia can help to raise awareness of those who interact with and/or care for individuals with this condition. Raised awareness has the potential for contributing to more effective advance planning for how to meet their present and future needs for personal and financial security, physical care, and emotional support (Agency for Health Care Policy and Research [AHCPR], 1996a).

"IT CAME TO THE POINT WHERE WE NEEDED A DIAGNOSIS."

Despite the advantages of early detection, there often is delay in seeking a professional evaluation of symptoms. Affected individuals usually are not the ones who take the initiative. Typically, family members or close friends influence or arrange for clinical assessment as they become aware of changes in persons' behaviors, personalities, or abilities to care for themselves, communicate, and manage daily life activities. As awareness dawns of a need to obtain definitive answers and professional assistance, flashes of hindsight over missed warning signs occur.

Daughter: "There were just a lot of clues that we really didn't put together until it came to the point where we needed a diagnosis. For example, he had lots of 'fender benders,' and it's amazing he didn't have more. He began to have trouble playing bridge. I had taken over paying the bills because Mom said, 'Something's wrong.' But it wasn't clear that we needed to do something until Mom went into the hospital, because she was the one who took care of everything. Then we realized that Mom needed help too."

In addition, persuading a person to agree to be evaluated is not always an easy or straightforward undertaking. Knowledge of the person and how to broach the subject and obtain cooperation is essential. Individuals who lack insight regarding others' concerns about them may bristle at perceived attempts to influence them and invade their privacy. Or the threat of discovery may be a problem for those who live in fear of embarrassment and/or commitment to an institution if others find out that all is not well with them. Underlying these concerns is the consideration that adults should be free to determine for themselves what is in their own best interests. Thus, an elder's resistance to seeking help in these circumstances may provoke moral distress in family and friends who feel a sense of responsibility and want to be of assistance. Sometimes neighbors and people without close attachments to individuals express relief when family members intervene but are otherwise reluctant to report their observations and concerns about a neighbor's or fellow community member's actions.

> *Daughter: "Some of the neighbors admitted to us that they were very glad she was going to get some help. They could probably see it more than we could. [For instance], it came out that they had seen her driving on the sidewalk."*

Diagnosis may be delayed or hindered when, through good intentions or for personal reasons, persons compensate for individuals in ways that obscure the extent of their impairments.

> *A daughter recalls: "I was encouraging her to move into an apartment because the house was getting to be too much for her. But no matter what I would say, she wasn't listening. She didn't want to leave her neighbor. Her neighbor would come every morning for coffee and she became very dependent on the help in the bathroom, help getting dressed. . . . Later, when she got worse, I think they were covering it up. We didn't know that until she got really bad. And one day I [discovered] that she was unable to get out of bed and dress herself."*

Spouses, in particular, may seek to protect one another and avoid separation. This can involve the unintentional collusion of other people in discounting symptomatic behavior.

For example, a daughter explains: "They were married for fifty years. They were very loyal and loved each other a great deal. She had a lot of depression but was never treated for it. And she would always lose stuff. But the difference with her losing stuff was that she believed that somebody else took it. And we kind of joked about it and thought she was a flake about some things. We didn't know it was an illness until it got very progressed because our dad hid it. When our father died, we knew we couldn't leave her alone. In fact, she had progressed so badly, we wonder if she knew he died."

People who come to evaluation when their disease is well advanced often do so precipitously, out of some crisis (e.g., loss of a critical caregiver, accident or injury) that makes it impossible for them to continue as before. These circumstances tend to add to everyone's distress. When persons refuse to be evaluated, their capacity to make an informed choice about the matter may be questioned. But forcing an evaluation in the absence of clear danger will not serve (Rabins et al., 1999, pp. 237–238).

A diagnosis of dementia requires evidence of decline from previous levels of functioning, and impairment in multiple cognitive domains (American Psychiatric Association 1994; Small et al., 1997). Documentation from a variety of sources is used to establish the diagnosis. Even if dementia is not present, this multifaceted evaluation is necessary to identify some other cause of symptoms (e.g., an undiagnosed medical condition, depression, drug interactions or side effects).

A comprehensive assessment (AHCPR, 1996b) involves a *focused history* that includes careful attention to: onset and progression of current symptoms; relevant diseases and disorders, including conditions that could contribute to cognitive impairment (e.g., infections, neurological problems, alcohol or substance abuse, exposure to environmental toxins, history of head trauma); family history of dementia or genetic conditions that lead to dementia (e.g., Huntington's disease); and medication history to assess for drugs associated with cognitive changes.

A *focused physical examination* will be needed to assess for conditions that cause delirium (e.g., some infections, hypoglycemia, adverse drug effects) and to rule out tumors and vascular lesions. These constitute medical emergencies that may coexist with or be mistaken for dementia and will require immediate treatment.

A *functional status evaluation* requires reliable informants to rate persons' abilities to perform a variety of daily tasks, such as shopping, preparing meals, keeping appointments, writing checks, and taking medications. The persons themselves should be asked first and informed that others will be interviewed. Depending on their relationship with the particular individual, family members or close friends may increase the accuracy of the information, especially if the person is experiencing memory loss or lacks insight regarding the severity of his/her decline.

Screening for depression is important because depression as the cause of memory loss, diminished ability to think or concentrate, fatigue, and change in appetite and sleep patterns may respond favorably to treatment. Diagnosis is difficult, however, because depression and dementia may be confused with one another or they may present together. Failure to treat persons with coexisting depression and dementia will add to the stress of the condition. However, antidepressants must be used appropriately and with caution because they also can worsen confusion in individuals with progressive dementia.

A *mental status assessment* lends an additional dimension to the clinical picture provided by the person's current symptoms and level of functional ability. There are several short tests used to screen for such things as short-term recall, aphasia (language impairment), apraxia (impaired ability to perform motor tasks such as writing), agnosia (impairment in pattern recognition), concentration, and spatial orientation. These tests do not establish the diagnosis and may not be as helpful as other sources of information in assessing mild dementia. However, they provide a useful baseline for evaluating the course of cognitive impairment across time and are needed as documentation of its suspected nature. (The presence of vision, hearing, and motor impairments will need to be taken into consideration when choosing, administering, and scoring tests. The extent to which other factors, such as older age, educational level, and culture influence test performance also must be weighed when interpreting the results of the testing.)

Laboratory testing may be considered in some cases (e.g., tests for anemia or vitamin deficiencies, thyroid studies, blood chemistry checks for diabetes, liver or kidney problems). Brain imaging may be used to rule specific conditions in or out. If this sort of additional information is needed, Computed Tomography (CT scan) often is sufficient. Magnetic Resonance Imaging (MRI) may help to identify changes in the brain that indicate a stroke or a tumor. Single Photon Emission Computed Tomography (SPECT) or Positron Emission Tomography (PET) are used to look for areas of compromised blood flow. However, these advanced radiologic techniques are not always necessary.

A *family assessment* includes information about the person's environment and those available to provide support and meet needs. It also is important to assess family members' insight into the person's condition and its prognosis, the extent to which they may need help, and the resources available to them. Examiners are expected to be alert for signs of abuse and neglect by caregivers, which they may be required by law to report. This matter needs to be approached sensitively, since persons with dementia also can be prone to falls and self-injury. Conversely, families need to understand that elder abuse is a serious social problem that cannot be ignored.

> *A daughter explains:* "We found her on the floor when we got there; and we think she tripped or toppled out of her chair. She was black and blue on her forehead, her nose, her chin and the side of her leg. The doctor asked her if somebody hit her. And I wondered, 'How could he ever have thought that?' I didn't really think about it [how others might view her appearance] until later. She told them she fell down the stairs, which wasn't so. If she had fallen down the stairs she would have broken bones. But we knew then that she needed all day care."

If evaluation establishes a diagnosis of dementia, follow-up efforts will turn toward identification of the disease process most likely responsible (differential diagnosis), assessment of the severity of functional and cognitive impairment, and description of other features for which treatment may be necessary (e.g., behavior, mood, or motor disturbances). Follow-up may involve repeating some tests to document stable or progressing cognitive problems or additional neuropsychological testing. The most common diseases that cause progressive dementia are Alzheimer's disease, involving the destruction of brain cells, and cerebrovascular disease, involving a series of strokes within the brain (multi-infarct/vascular dementias). Dementia due to Lewy body disease (characterized by microscopic abnormalities in the brain) occurs less frequently. Its symptoms are similar to Alzheimer's disease with the addition of mild symptoms of Parkinson's disease occurring early in the illness (e.g., walking difficulties due to stiffness, slowness, and poor balance). Pick's disease is a rare form of slowly progressive dementia involving loss of brain tissue. The cause of the disease is unknown (National Institute of Neurological Disorders and Stroke, 2001). Also HIV- or AIDS-associated dementia (also called AIDS dementia complex) has become a more noticeable phenomenon over the last decade, with brain infection caused by HIV itself (Price, 1998). Although associated with a poor prognosis and rapid decline, the advent of multiple drug therapy has slowed progression of this type of dementia, estimated to be present in approximately 10–15% of persons with HIV infection or AIDS (Sellers & Angerame, 2002). There are many other forms of dementia, as well. However, it is not uncommon for the clinical findings to reflect atypical patterns that prevent the precise identification of a pathological cause. (See Rabins et al., 1999, for a more detailed discussion of diseases and conditions causing different patterns of dementia.)

Families for whom confirmation of the diagnosis was the primary reason for the evaluation visit, and those for whom return visits pose a hardship (e.g., traveling distance or uncooperative family member), do not always pursue specialized follow-up testing. Therefore, clinicians usually will raise the relevant issues that they know families must face in days to come at the visit when the diagnosis is made. These include the person's competence to drive a car and perform other activities that raise safety issues; execution of a durable power of attorney and health care proxy; and living arrangements that will provide adequate support and supervision. They may prescribe one of the drugs available to treat symptoms of cognitive deterioration. Although these will not halt the progression of the disease or make a difference in every case, medication may enable some people with mild or moderate dementia to function better for a brief period of time (National Institute on Aging, 1997). Even if this does not happen or provides only a slight reprieve, there is the knowledge that an attempt to slow the progress of the disease has been made. In any case, the individual's primary physician needs to receive a complete report and recommendations.

"SHE FOUGHT ME TOOTH AND NAIL."

The conventional wisdom is to try to relocate persons with dementia who live alone to a more protective environment where, possibly, they can make friends, be closer to family members, and get used to a new place before the illness makes adaptation harder. Some individuals are ready or can be persuaded to make a move. But there are many who do not want to leave their homes. Personal daily routines are easier to carry out in this familiar environment. Ties to people and daily rhythms of the neighborhood can be soothing and reassuring. Initially, people may appear more oriented in this setting. And, perhaps remaining in one's own home fosters a belief that nothing will change. Therefore, it can be quite shocking when changes eventually come, often uninvited. For example, it may be alarming when family members with helpful intentions invade the person's domain. Families with plans of putting the household in order are not always prepared to have their efforts rebuffed. But for homeowners, the takeover of their territory and possessions can be very threatening. Appeals to reason will fail in the face of fear and lack of insight.

Daughter: "She fought me tooth and nail. The accumulation of papers and things! Furniture and rugs ruined from incontinence! When we went into the house and I saw what was happening I said, 'This can't go on. I've got to come in here and start straightening out.' And her words were, 'Mind your own business. This is my house, not yours; and I can live like this if I want to.' I said, 'I don't believe this. I'm your daughter!' But I don't think she ever forgave me for stepping in; and I can't tell you what I threw away on her. I bet I threw out things I shouldn't have. It just got to the point where it was absolutely overwhelming."

Individuals who are accustomed to living alone and being very independent often have difficulty adjusting to lifestyle changes that result from families assuming more responsibility for their safety and well-being. Their vehement protests when matters are taken out of their hands may come as a surprise.

A daughter recalls: "We started checking up on her. Sometimes she was agreeable to it. Sometimes she'd be a little annoyed and say, 'Don't you think I can take care of myself?' And it was not like Mom to be like that. There was a rudeness that we sensed. But when we took away her medications . . . ! Mom never swore. But what she called us! I didn't know Mom knew those words. We were yelled at because we finally had to make the decision. She was mad about the interference; but I'm sure she was overdosing. I said, 'I'll bring them to you every morning now,' and that's what I did."

It can be especially difficult for caregivers to take away things that are closely involved with an individual's sense of identity and independence. One of the earliest of these crisis points occurs when a person is unsafe to drive a car but is unwilling to stop. If persuasion fails, the family may have to take the keys, dispose of the car, or disable it in some way that renders it temporarily unusable. Some find this difficult to do.

Son: "I really did not understand Alzheimer's disease. I realized she would get lost; and I refused to ride in the car with her. I remember one day we were meeting for lunch and I arrived first. Pretty soon horns were honking, tires were screeching, and I looked. And sure enough, here she came, down the middle of the road. At that point she was lining up the crease of the hood of the car with the center line. But at the time, it was easier not to say anything to avoid the battle that would result from it. My mother was very determined, very stubborn, and she was going to do things her way."

Families may use an indirect approach to avoid a personal confrontation. The physician or county caseworker may volunteer to be "the bad guy" who says that it is time to stop driving. States have different policies about license renewals that might provide a creative way out. And excuses may serve, such as cars that need repairs indefinitely. Seeking to prevent the person from being injured in an accident is not the only reason for being concerned. Ultimately, the decision to become involved and take action is a matter of public safety for which family members bear responsibility if they know that the person poses a risk.

> *Daughter: "That's a dangerous issue. I see that as a real weak spot with a lot of people that don't have the courage or the nerve to take the car away. I was crying, 'How can I do that to my mother? You know what she'll be like without a car.' My husband said, 'What if she kills a child? How would you feel then?' That was all I had to hear."*

There is little consensus on when driving privileges should be revoked. And, laws about reporting persons to motor vehicle bureaus differ by state. Rabins et al. (1999) recommend that anyone who has received a diagnosis of dementia should stop driving and be evaluated prior to a decision about resuming this activity (p. 239). The ADRDA policy statement on driving and dementia (2001b) states, in part: "(1) A diagnosis of Alzheimer's disease is not, on its own, a sufficient reason to withdraw driving privileges. The determining factor . . . should be an individual's driving ability . . . (2) If there is concern that an individual with Alzheimer's disease has impaired driving ability, and the person would like to continue driving, a formal assessment of driving skills should be administered. One type of assessment is an on-the-road driving evaluation by trained personnel. Such an assessment should lead to specific recommendations, consistent with state laws and regulations, as to whether the individual is able to drive and with what restrictions (if any). (3) Physicians and other health professionals, public safety officials and state regulatory agencies are encouraged to address the issue of driving safety with individuals with Alzheimer's disease and their families. . . . Physicians and families must decide in the best interests of the individual whose decision-making capacity is impaired. (4) Further research is needed to identify optimal methods for physicians and licensing bureaus to identify impaired drivers and, when necessary, to withdraw driving privileges in a manner that preserves the dignity of the individual with Alzheimer's disease . . . "

Taking over management of the person's finances and decision-making functions can be equally anxiety provoking for everyone. It is better if plans have been put in place before a transfer of responsibility becomes necessary, but people often delay. Families may find it awkward to discuss legal and financial matters, health care proxies, and funeral arrangements with persons who seem well and are still managing their own affairs, and so they procrastinate. Also, some individuals raise obstacles by being very secretive about their personal affairs, but it is important to attend to these concerns while they still are able to grasp the basic issues and give consent. Engaging the services of a lawyer knowledgeable in these areas and in the particular laws of the state in which the person resides is a wise thing to do. This advice is germane to all family members including spouses, who will need to be sure they are legally positioned to assume decision making responsibilities for the person with dementia and oversee joint property and resources as he/she becomes increasingly less able to do so.

In addition to help with estate planning and a will, a lawyer needs to draw up a *durable* power of attorney (POA). The document must indicate that this power to transact business on the person's behalf will not be affected by his/her physical or mental incapacity. Specific powers include management of finances, securities and investments, real estate, personal property, taxes, and, in some states, authorization of medical care and treatment. It is important that these matters are taken care of while the person still is able to understand the purpose of the document he/she is signing (the issue of competency).

Daughter: "We did this while she was still pretty much 'with it'. She was forgetting a lot of things. But she still knew she had money. And we talked about if she was sick we would need some papers saying we could use her money to pay her bills."

Persons also should be encouraged to appoint a health care proxy/ surrogate to make medical decisions for them if they become incapacitated. This person can but does not have to be the one who holds the power of attorney. Each state has its own advance directive forms that provide a legal mechanism for specifying who the health care proxy will be, as well as medical treatments that individuals do or do not wish to receive in the event that they lose the ability to make decisions for themselves. Some states call this latter directive (about specific treatment wishes) a living will. These witnessed forms allow persons to designate their wishes about treatments that they have strong feelings about receiving or not receiving if they are in a terminal condition or state of permanent unconsciousness (e.g., cardiac resuscitation, mechanical respiration, feeding tubes, intravenous infusions, surgery, renal dialysis, antibiotics). If it is possible that a person could be receiving care in a state other than the one in which he/she lives, it is advisable to obtain and fill out forms for both states. Persons are encouraged to give photocopies of the signed originals to their surrogate, doctor, family, close friends, clergy, and anyone else who might be involved in their health care. The declaration also should be a part of the medical record in the event of hospitalization or admission to a nursing home or alternative care facility. (These forms may not be effective in the event of a medical emergency. Ambulance personnel in some states are required to perform cardiopulmonary resuscitation unless they are given a separate order signed by a physician that directs otherwise. Interested persons should speak to their physicians, since not all states have laws authorizing these "nonhospital do-not-resuscitate orders.") Advance directive forms for specific states are available through a national not-for-profit organization called Partnership for Caring. Persons with dementia should be encouraged to participate in decisions about their care by talking about their wishes concerning medical treatment often, and particularly as their medical condition changes.

Families sometimes discover that persons are actively interested in making their own funeral plans. As difficult as it may be for others, this is an opportunity to help individuals for whom this is important to obtain the satisfaction of putting their affairs in order. Organizing information for their obituary or memorials can be a celebration of their lifetime accomplishments. Those who express less interest still should be asked tactfully about their wishes, prior arrangements, and the location of needed documents. (The Veterans Health Administration will provide perpetual care of a grave site for a veteran and spouse in a military cemetery. Veterans Administration social workers and also funeral directors can arrange for this well in advance.)

Community services help extend the length of time that people can be sustained safely in their own homes. However, persons must be willing to receive help. Sometimes individuals are reluctant to accept meals or allow an aide to assist them with self-care, errands, or light housekeeping for a couple of hours or so a week. Pride, lack of insight that help is needed, and fear of the unknown all may be factors. If individuals cannot be persuaded, agencies will not force them to receive assistance. But fears about strangers coming into the home often can be overcome. Negotiating how they may be able to help then depends on the relationship that follows. Professional helpers are trained to interact with elderly people with dementia and most are very skillful in what they do, becoming an important part of the support network. The potential for difficulties with aides who are unacceptable or unreliable needs to be evaluated and reported. The retained abilities of persons with dementia can be greatly enhanced by their acceptance of even a minimal number of services. Some strong-willed or reclusive individuals with a long history of resisting offers of help may pose a challenge.

Daughter: "We knew she wasn't eating properly, so we tried to encourage Meals On Wheels because we thought one good meal a day would do it. We knew she could make coffee in the morning and maybe some toast or something. But she absolutely refused. Friends suggested we just sign her up for it. But we knew what would happen if they came to the door because it's happened before. She'd toss people out."

Persons should not be forced to move unless there is clear evidence of danger. An experienced community-based caseworker may prove to be a strong family ally in winning their confidence and phasing in support services. If there are questions about an individual's ability to live alone, a professional evaluation may be necessary.

Day programs can help to relieve family caregivers while offering care and socialization to the individual. In-home aide services also become increasingly important as functional and cognitive abilities continue to decline. Over time, it becomes less and less possible to leave persons with dementia unattended. Some reasons for this include immobilizing passivity, incontinence, short attention span and poor judgment that put them at risk for accidents (e.g., cooking on an open flame), or a tendency to wander. Wandering is a frequently encountered problem that can take different forms, from simple meandering or intense pacing to attempting to get away. Persons may be trying to go somewhere (like the bathroom), lose their sense of direction, and forget what it was that they wanted to do. They may be bored and restless, not feeling well, reacting to a negative stimulus (e.g., anxiety over showering/bathing), confused by changes in their environment, or more disoriented as nighttime approaches. Sometimes looking to discover and relieve the cause (e.g., pain), tolerance, gentle reassurance, walking with them, or providing alternative activities will help. Solutions will be dependent on possible reasons for the behavior. Medication may help, as a last resort, since drug side effects also can make symptoms worse. Sometimes there is nothing beyond calm reassurance and provision of a safe environment that will counteract this result of brain disease. Families will need help when wandering is a problem. Ultimately, this may be the symptom that ends their ability to maintain persons in their home environments.

Sister: "*We went from four-hour care, to eight-hour care, to twelve-hour care, to twenty-four-hour care. But it got to the point that even the aides that were coming in couldn't handle him. He was a big man, and he'd just walk out the door when he felt like it. If they'd try to redirect him, he'd say, 'You're not going to tell me what to do.' They couldn't stop him. And I was trying to manage all this from a distance.*"

The Alzheimer's Association Safe Return Program assists in the safe return of persons with dementia who wander and become lost. The ADRDA Safe Return Fact Sheet (2002) describes it as "a nationwide identification, support, and registration program working at the community level . . . Assistance is available 24 hours, every day, whenever a person is lost or found. Estimates are that nearly 60% of the 4 million people with Alzheimer's disease will wander . . . There is no way to predict when wandering may occur . . . If not located within 24 hours, 46% will die, succumbing to hypothermia or dehydration . . . Safe Return has over 68,000 people registered nationally . . . [and] a nearly 100% recovery rate [compared to a] less than 50% safe return of nonregistered people who wander."

Live-in companions can provide relief when demands for assistance and supervision are reasonably modest. But they may not be able to manage upsetting behaviors that can occur. Persons with dementia sometimes develop ideas that people are taking things from them, conspiring against or intending to harm them. It may be the result of disorientation, lessened ability to understand and cope with ordinary daily events, or misinterpretation of others' attempts to assist them. They may be struggling with confusing feelings about what is happening to them. Or they may be suffering from frightening hallucinations or delusions.

Son: "*We hired a woman that we knew to come and live with her; and she lasted three months. She couldn't take it anymore. Mom began to carry a butcher knife around. We had to go and take it away from her.*"

"IT WAS TRAUMATIC FOR HER AND FOR US."

Lasting patience is required in interactions with persons who have dementia. They may direct their anger and frustration toward family and others; mistakenly accuse them of stealing from them, lying to them, or not informing them of things; use poor judgment; behave inappropriately; call constantly, or demand more attention at times than friends and family members are able to give. They cannot control these behaviors. And the deterioration of their abilities to manage their lives, their relationships, and their emotions is stressful and painful to watch. Therefore, family members need to recognize signs of fatigue and strain in their own relationships with the person and with others.

For example, a daughter-in-law says: "It was traumatic for her and for us. One minute you get so angry at her, and the next minute you want to try to reason with her. But I've read all the literature that says you can't reason with persons who have dementia. You should try to go along with them. My husband wouldn't accept that; and he would try to reason with her. So that would upset her; and it would cause tension between the two of us."

Interactions among family members may be strained. Families respond differently to the challenges of caring for the person with dementia. Of course, some persons do not have families to care for them. Or family members may be too ill, unable, or unwilling to become involved. But there are many more instances in which families who are available, locally or far away, struggle to find ways to maintain and support individuals. Sometimes illness brings family members together, causing them to bridge geographic distance and put aside past differences to work collaboratively on behalf of the person who needs their help. At other times, old conflicts are resurrected or new ones arise over opposing opinions about decisions that must be made. There also may be ill feelings if members feel that some are not assuming their share of the caregiving burden. Problems often stem from lack of understanding about the nature of dementia and how it shapes present care concerns and future actions. At times the learning needs of family members who have had less contact and involvement with the person pose challenges to caregivers who are most familiar with the situation and have borne the major responsibility.

A local caregiver recalls friction among his siblings, who lived out of state, over decisions regarding their mother's care: "They quarreled over where she was to go, and this thing and that thing. One wanted to take her home, the other wanted her to move to a place in the city. I was the one who had been taking care of her all these years; and I told her she was in charge of what she wanted to do. It was a big argument, and I was in the middle. But I stayed out of it and just kept taking care of what had to be taken care of. And after they went home I moved her to [an assisted living facility]. But I also bought a book [about caring for elders with dementia] and sent it to my brother, because you can't talk to him. He called and said, 'Somebody sent me this book.' And I said, 'No kidding! Really? What's it about?' Well, he'd read it; and I [confirmed that] this is what [caring for someone with dementia] is all about. After that everything calmed down in the family."

"THERE WAS NO WAY WE COULD LET HER LIVE ALONE."

The rate at which dementia progresses and how it affects people's cognitive and functional capacities is highly variable. Therefore, it is difficult to judge how long it may be possible to enable individuals diagnosed with this condition to remain alone in their own homes. Stages of dementia have been described as mild, moderate, and severe. But they tend to overlap, and not all persons with dementia have the same symptoms.

People with mild dementia will be able to carry on most of their usual activities unsupervised. This stage is said to last for two to four years, blending into the moderate stage that may last from two to eight years. Thus, some people do very well over a relatively long period of time with support and assistance that compensates for their fluctuating abilities. The fact that there are fluctuations, with people having "good days" as well as not-so-good days is important to bear in mind. Not only does it create hope on the not-so-good days for a better day tomorrow, but it should serve to focus attention on retained abilities, which may be many.

First noted changes tend to be increased difficulty with retention of information and short-term memory, use of language (e.g., forgetting names of people and common objects), and difficulty with written expression and other higher level functions (e.g., balancing a check-book). Judgment may be impaired under some circumstances. This is part of the controversy over when people with dementia should stop driving. Habitual driving skills may be intact, and if individuals are encountering no difficulties, some believe they should be allowed to continue until problems are observed. However, driving is a complex skill calling for quick, accurate decisions in unexpected or confusing situations. Reaction time and judgment are important criteria to consider. Perceptual difficulties also have been receiving attention for the role they may play. Researchers believe that "getting lost" while driving may not represent simply forgetting where one is, but an inability to perceive and interpret multiple visual cues that most people absorb and process without being consciously aware of them (O'Brien et al., 2001; Tetewsky & Duffy, 1999). A goal in studying this phenomenon and perhaps developing more sophisticated tests for perceptual difficulties is increased accuracy in determining how long people may be considered safe to retain the mobility and independence that driving a car represents. This is not a small matter, since depression and strong emotional reactions brought about by unnecessarily restraining and depriving people of the means to pursue their normal activities only will worsen the situation. People with mild to moderate dementia need respect and latitude to continue doing everything that they can do safely, without interference. This is a valuable time for families to enjoy the present in every way possible, to celebrate what persons are able to do, and to plan for the future (i.e., designate power of attorney and health care proxy; make decisions about when to turn over various personal and financial matters).

Later changes involve increased confusion and anxiety along with forgetting how to perform ordinary daily activities. Safety concerns become more of an issue.

For example, a daughter recalls: "One thing that frightened me to death was she called me up one day and said, 'I can't figure out how to turn off the stove.' So I went up there and she had every single burner on the stove on; and that scared me. That really scared me. Then we got her a microwave. We thought it would be easier. Of course, she couldn't figure out how to use that either. So we thought she'd be fine at Greystone Hall [pseudonym] because she wouldn't have to get meals and they'd kind of watch out for her, being a proprietary home. There was no way we could let her live alone."

Self-care abilities begin to decline. There is difficulty with simple ordinary tasks like getting dressed, bathing, or going to the toilet. Persons may not know what to do with food that is provided or may forget to eat.

Daughter: "We went through this: 'I don't know what's the matter with you people. I don't need help.' . . . 'Well, you do, Mom, because you haven't been eating. And the doctor says you're losing weight.' . . . 'Well, he doesn't know what he's talking about. I have been eating regular meals.' . . . 'No, Mom, you haven't been eating regular meals.' . . . 'Well, yes I have.' So I said to my brother, 'You're going to have to get involved in this. You've been the favorite in this family all our life, and you're the only one she'll listen to. So he finally said, 'Mom, I think you're going to have to go someplace.' "

As mentioned earlier, wandering may become an issue. And, for some individuals, loss of balance and falls begin to increase.

> *Daughter: "She fell and broke a hip, got rehab, fell again and damaged the same hip. Rehab took longer that time and she never really was quite herself after that. Then she was falling more and more, and I think her mind was getting more confused."*

Previously successful systems for administration of medications begin to fail.

> *Daughter: "He had a container for the pills [with a compartment for each day of the week] that I would fill. But the next day I would find it would be dumped out all over the shelf."*

As symptoms mount, families may start exploring residential care options. There are an increasing number and variety of types of senior housing, proprietary homes, and assisted living facilities. Some of these may be designed to meet special needs of persons with dementia. Thus, many individuals have had experiences in alternative living situations before they are admitted to a nursing home.

"I DON'T THINK THEY WATCHED HER VERY WELL."

Community-based alternative living facilities are not all equally staffed and organized to manage certain symptoms associated with dementia. Some will not be able to care for individuals with more than mild incontinence problems. There may not be adequate supervision for people who fall frequently. And many are not able to reliably monitor persons who are prone to wander outside of the facility.

> *A son recalls: "The adult home was all right [but] I don't think they watched her very well. I really don't. She got out one night, and I got a call—'Your mother got out tonight.' Well, how the heck did she get out? Those doors are supposed to be secure aren't they? Because that was one thing I asked—'Is this a secure area?' [I was told], 'Yes.' Okay. Well, they found her walking down the road. The police picked her up at two o'clock in the morning . . . in her nightclothes. I was ready to blow my stack, and I went up and told them what I thought. 'Well, you know she has dementia,' they said."*

There is a perception that senior housing communities and assisted living situations are more structured and secure than they really are. Indeed, they may offer more services and amenities than can be provided for persons living alone in the community. Thus, they can serve as a temporary solution for meeting the increasing needs of some persons with dementia. They may offer relief from certain household duties (e.g., meal preparation, laundry, cleaning); limited surveillance (e.g., daily checks on people by hall monitors, emergency call buttons, staff on premises); various opportunities for socialization (e.g., programs/activities, clubs, worship services, social gatherings); and specialized services (e.g., transportation, hair salon, library, fitness center). Some facilities offer select health care options, such as medication administration or health professionals on call. However, there always will be a potential for tension between the actual care needs of specific individuals and the limits of the package offered by the facility. When personal care needs exceed the service package, the facilities are not able to accept the associated risks.

> *For example, a daughter explains: "She would go out, walk around in the mall down the street and do what she wanted. And then she would stroll back in when she was done; and they'd just be going crazy looking for her. But the thing that really pushed it was that a few times the director had to go out in her car and look for my mother. People would say they'd seen her walking down the middle of the road [and she would approach strangers on the street or in the mall]. So they just refused to have her there anymore unless she had a 24-hour aide. Well, she couldn't afford that, and, besides, she hated it. She hated to have somebody next to her all the time. So then we started looking around for a place that would take someone who was a 'wanderer', which is what Mother was called even though I'm sure she knew just where she was going."*

There also may be an inherent conflict between goals of assisted living designed to promote independence and the growing dependency needs of persons with dementia. Families sometimes find that meeting the person's needs for more structure is in contradiction to the value of personal autonomy that is promoted by the facility as a primary tenet of community life.

> *Daughter: "Fellworth Manor [pseudonym] built a new wing that they said was going to be for [people with] dementia. So that's where I ended up putting him, and I would spend every Saturday with him. When he first got there, it seemed to be okay, but then he did get lost. And I'm sure that*

he was inappropriately crossing the street, which made me very nervous. Today the residents have rights, so they could not keep him in. And he was buying beer, [that is a dependency problem for him and is known to increase his risk of falling]. I spent some time talking to the gentleman at the liquor store, who said that was fine. They have refused to allow certain persons to buy. But the [grocery store] wouldn't help me out at all. So that was a constant worry. It is so hard to find places."

Persons in alternative living situations still are members of the larger community and retain all the freedom and privileges to which they have been accustomed. When there is a question of needing to set limits on their behavior or when they do not fit the profile of the majority of people living in the facility, families may find that some previously faced challenges of community living remain unchanged.

"WE DECIDED TO MOVE IN WITH HER."

Many persons with dementia are cared for at home by spouses and/or other family members. "Home" may be their own place of residence or they may come to live in the primary caregiver's home. In either case, families will find that the number of hours devoted to meeting the person's needs as well as the physical and emotional toll of those efforts increase over time. Sometimes the personal price is more than can be endured.

Son: "She would wander, and we started getting phone calls from the police. That's when we decided to move in with her. It was not fun. It was not pleasant. It lasted three months, and then I couldn't take it anymore. I couldn't come home from work and deal with that every day. Things were hidden, and she'd burn things up in the oven . . . or have the table set for twenty people. It was just a lot of stress. And then [it was difficult] to sleep at night when you knew she was wandering around downstairs and could burn up the house."

Whether or not in-home family caregiving is manageable and beneficial is situation dependent. Some symptoms of the disease are more difficult to cope with than others, even when there is additional assistance to provide occasional relief. Increased nocturnal activity, lack of cooperation, belligerence, and attempts to escape that risk potential harm make care at home challenging and threaten others' health and well-being.

Daughter: "*She would get up two and three times at night and dress and undress. And we had a monitor in our room so I would hear her. I'd be up all night because she was up and down and up and down. And she would be quite belligerent if you tried to talk to her and say it's the middle of the night and she should go back to bed. She'd hallucinate, and we were frightened she would walk out the front door. We just couldn't supervise her 24 hours a day, 7 days a week, even with the aides coming in to feed and help her in the morning. It only takes her about one minute, and she's on the go. And she can really move fast.*"

Caregivers typically face multiple demands that compete for their time and energy, including family and employment obligations. Those who themselves are elderly and/or in ill health are at a further disadvantage. And limited finances also create strains by precluding some fee for service care options. The assistance of community agencies, such as local offices on aging and national or local branches of the Alzheimer's Association, can help guide individuals to accessible supportive services. But they cannot remove the burden of responsibility that always accompanies decisions to provide care at home for persons with dementia.

"I WANTED TO MAKE EVERYTHING RIGHT, AND YOU JUST CAN'T."

Some family caregivers bear up well and perceive that they and the person being cared for share a mutual benefit in their ability to keep him/her at home with them for as long as possible. This may add precious years to their time together, making any sacrifice or hardship seem worthwhile. Other people often marvel at the caregiver's devotion and fortitude. However, it is dangerous and unfair to hold up such an example as a model of what families can or ought to do. Every person's experience with dementia is unique to him/herself; and family circumstances are equally unique. A difficult situation can be made more so when families feel that they are somehow lacking if they cannot maintain their family member at home as well or as long as they think others do or as they think they should. Thoughtful reassessment of options will be needed if caregiving becomes injurious to caregivers' health, jeopardizes relationships with and responsibilities toward others, and/or threatens livelihoods. It is wise to know one's limits because in extreme cases, severe frustration and desperate measures to cope on the part of caregivers can disintegrate into abuse and neglect of the person with dementia.

This represents a set of circumstances to be alert for and to guard against.

Although home care can work well, at least for awhile, it should be accepted that it is not the best choice for everybody. However, the guilt and suffering associated with the thought of pursuing any other option can be enormous for some people. Part of this may be because one of the dilemmas of caring for a family member with dementia is that it is not purely a matter of logic and knowing what the options are. It is an emotional and spiritual journey across a surreal landscape in the company of a person so familiar and yet so changed that what seems to be happening cannot be taken in all at one time.

> *A wife recalls: "You try to make them as normal as possible, and so if he'd say, 'I don't know how. What do you want me to do?' I would say, 'You know how to do that. You've done it all your life.' And I'd get very angry with him. Then I would calm down and try to show him how. And, you know, for a few minutes he could do it; and then he couldn't. I honestly don't know what was going through my head at the time. I just know I had to have been very angry. I didn't want what was happening to happen. I wanted to try to make everything right, and you just can't. I was giving him total care when we started the nursing home search. He couldn't feed, or bathe, or dress himself, or go to the bathroom. And there were times when he would try to hit me just because he was frustrated. That was kind of scary. For awhile he understood what I was saying to him, although he could not talk to me. But then when that stopped, it was very difficult. And [through it all] I was just trying to make life as normal as possible. I think it was denial of a sort. Back then I would have said, 'Oh, no. I've accepted it.' But you try so hard because you just don't want this to be happening. I think I was in total denial [of] the fact that I was losing the person that I knew. You know, he's no longer there, although he looks just the same."*

"I FELT LIKE I'D BE BETRAYING HIM."

Evaluating the appropriateness of continuing to maintain persons with dementia at home is not always straightforward. In particular, families may experience uncertainty when moments of confusion and inability to function alternate with periods of lucidity during which the person is able to make decisions, communicate, and function effectively. It is not clear why failing brains seem to rebound from time to time. But it is important to understand that this is a phenomenon over which the individual absolutely has no control. The corresponding effect on family members is one of low points and high points. At the low points, strength threatens to desert them and spirits drop with the weight of their impending loss of the person they knew. But at unexpected high points, when the individual seems most like he/she was before, there may be a surge of excitement and relief over this rekindling of the former self. The high points make it hard to think about nursing home admission. But, eventually, this decision may have to be faced.

When the individual is known to have expressed fears about being in a nursing home, the decision to override his/her wishes often is accompanied by painful guilt.

> *A wife recalls: "He was wandering outdoors at night. I had to call the police to look for him. Then he started to become incontinent, and finally I had more than I could handle. All this was piling up on me [but] I kept him. . . . Well, he was like that probably about five-six months at least; and it just got progressively worse. But I just didn't feel like I wanted to do it. I felt like I'd be betraying him. Then my family and friends said, 'You've got to think of your health so you'll be there for him.' I thought I was doing well, but other people could see [I was not]. So it was just something that I had to do; and I felt just terrible doing it. But I just couldn't take it anymore. He had said, 'I never want to go into a nursing home.' So I never said this was a nursing home. He thinks he's in a hospital. And every so often he'll say, 'Well, I'll only be here another month; and when I feel good and the weather turns, I've got to come home because I've got to take care of the tractor and I've got to take care of the yard.' And then I go home and feel so bad."*

The situation is complicated further by concerns over past promises that families may find they can no longer keep. Families anticipate a normal aging process for elders that they think they can accommodate. Disease is not part of this norm and dementia is a disease process that is not a part of normal aging. Thus, when disease happens, plans have to be reconfigured. For the family that has staunchly promised to support aging parents at home, the nursing home can represent failure, shame, and abandonment.

> *Daughter: "I promised my mother she would never go into a nursing home. I promised her I would never do anything like this. And did I keep my promise? No, I went back on it, didn't I? And my mother always knew she could depend on my word. [My doctor] said, 'Look, you've been a good mother; you've been a good wife; and a . . . [tearfully] and . . . a good*

daughter. What more can you do? It's time for you . . . It's time for you.'
This is what he told me."

"IT'S BROUGHT US CLOSE TOGETHER."

Living with dementia is a shared experience. Others whose lives the person with dementia touches also are part of his/her journey through illness. And, despite any stressful event's potential to produce instances of divisiveness, the possibilities of it bringing individuals together can be a source of reassurance. For family members, this sometimes involves long-distance commutes and communication as well as developing new roles and responsibilities.

For example, one family member relates: "The wonderful part of this is that it's brought us [the family] very close together. After years apart . . . and [each with our]different personalities . . . we've [been able to]research and plan together what would be best for her. We keep in touch. And I am thrilled with what [local family members] have done for Mom. It has helped me, being so far away, [because] when you're not the caregiver, there is a lot of guilt."

Persons with dementia retain their individuality in the eyes of family members and others who know them, even when some things about their lives and personalities come to reside less in actuality and more in others' memories. Sometimes there are memories of conflicted relationships with a parent, sibling, or spouse. But those memories said to comfort and sustain family members are ones that call to mind valued characteristics and cherished personal traits.

Daughter: "The most important thing about my mother is that she was very independent [and] very hard working. . . . She was the assistant foreman. (In those days women didn't get jobs as foremen. She helped train three guys who became foremen. Can you believe it?) . . . She [also] loved to have a good time . . . [Our] friends would come over . . . and we would have a lot of fun together [with her], laughing, and being silly . . . "

Wife: "The most endearing part of him was the way he laughed. He just enjoyed things so much. It took a lot to rile him; and no matter where he went, he had a big smile on his face. That was him—his big smile; and everybody said that about him too . . . He [also] took care of [his grandson] from the time he was six months old (because he had already retired); and they were so good together. They used to chat and talk like two little old men . . . One of my most vivid memories is of the two of them sitting out on our patio chatting away together."

Son: *"She'd buy bundles and bundles of yarn. And then she'd sit there and knit slippers and gloves. And she'd give them to the Salvation Army. . . . So that kept her busy. She was always doing for everybody else. She was the type of person [that] if she could help you out . . . [or] if you needed something, she'd be there."*

Some grieve what they describe as the "loss" or "death" of the person that they knew. But, even so, memories that predate the dementia are the taken-for-granted essence of who the person still is and always will be for family, even as they struggle to adjust to changes in abilities, moods, habits, and social behaviors influenced by his/her illness.

Families describe assessing the person with dementia's situation at any point in time as a balancing act. Alertness for signs of inability to function in various capacities needs to be tempered with appreciation for abilities that remain intact. It helps to avoid upsetting the routines that have served the person well. For example, self-care rituals and idiosyncratic patterns used to organize an individual's daily life may provide a comfort zone that persons can maintain well into dementia. Resisting the urge to correct and overlooking memory lapses and difficulties with spoken language also help to maintain the person's confidence and self-esteem. Families learn that it is important not to make assumptions about how much or what types of care a person with dementia may need. The goal should be to sustain and promote retained abilities and to compensate only for those that are failing. However, these efforts on the behalf of the person with dementia require extreme vigilance with changing circumstances. And the effort required in this undertaking should not be underestimated. Therefore, families need to think about resources to assure that they are not alone in this endeavor.

Although the person with dementia increasingly is in need of care and support, family members have similar needs to care for themselves. In order to do this effectively, they need information and guidance, encouragement, substantive assistance, and time out to preserve and restore physical and mental health. Community resources on aging and local chapters of the Alzheimer's Association can fulfill many needs for information and guidance. With the support of such agencies, families can seek out options that may help to ease their situation (e.g., in-home assistance, support groups, day and respite care). There also are helpful books that contain practical tips on caring for family members with dementia. *The 36-Hour Day* (Mace & Rabins, 1999) is one of the best known guides for families. The need for caregivers to care for themselves often is the most neglected as family members struggle to keep ill elders at home. Others' urgings may be necessary to raise the consideration that the well-being of the person with dementia and the well-being of family caregivers are related.

POSTSCRIPT

The Alzheimer's Disease and Related Disorders Association (ADRDA) is a national voluntary organization with over 70 area chapters and 2,000 support groups. It funds research, promotes public awareness, advocates legislation for persons with dementia and their families, and provides support services through its national, chapter, and volunteer network. It also publishes many helpful brochures on a variety of topics (e.g., fact sheets; caregiving advice; tips on communicating and interacting with persons with dementia; guidance on understanding legal and financial issues; steps to ensure safety; and signs of caregiver stress to watch for and address).

The Alzheimer's Disease Education and Referral Center (ADEAR Center) is a service of the National Institute on Aging, established in 1990 under provisions of the Alzheimer's Disease and Related Services Research Act of 1986. The ADEAR Center provides information and publications on Alzheimer's disease for health professionals, people with Alzheimer's disease and their families, and the public. It serves as a national resource for information on diagnosis, treatment issues, care issues and caregiver needs, long-term care, education, research, and ongoing programs. It also provides referrals to national and state resources, such as treatment centers, support groups, and family support services.

2

The Nursing Home Experience

OVERVIEW

This chapter begins with family member recollections of decisions to pursue nursing home admission. First, it focuses on organizational features and institutional policies that families exploring the options for persons with dementia may want to consider and it discusses changes in family member roles—from direct caregivers to advocates. Second, resident perspectives of what living in a nursing home is like are examined. Third, reflections on history, current challenges, and the place of nursing homes in long-term care seek to provide some context for resident issues and concerns.

Choosing to live in a nursing home is a serious life-altering decision. Others often must make the choice on behalf of the person with dementia. As cognitive impairment worsens and needs mount over time, maintaining caregiving networks for those who live alone becomes too difficult. And, similarly, providing care for family members at home becomes too challenging for caregivers. Indeed, as the physical and emotional demands on caregivers increase, their own health may decline more rapidly than the care receiver's health, placing both in jeopardy. However, even when caregivers sense that the risks to the individual are too great and/or that they themselves are reaching the limits of their endurance, the decision often is a hard-to-face turning point in everyone's lives.

I REMEMBER THINKING "THIS JUST IS HAPPENING TOO FAST."

Some families begin systematic exploration of nursing home options in advance. Others wait until further delay is no longer feasible.

For example, a wife recalls: "I'd never been here [nursing home] because we decided not to look at homes until we got the call [about an available bed]; and I remember thinking then, 'I don't know what I'm doing. This is just happening too fast.' But that's the best way to do it. And it was just like a load had been taken off my shoulders. I knew he was going to be cared for. I knew he was going to be fine. And whereas I was lonely, I didn't have to worry about him anymore."

Still others experience periods of uncertainty as their assessments of the person's situation and their own ability to cope with it fluctuate from day to day. In the following example, uncertainty, accompanied by a growing sense of the caregiver's need for relief, is complicated by the person's failure to meet the nursing home's admission criteria.

"This woman [from my support group] calls me all the time. She is in the process of getting her husband into a nursing home, but he can still do things for himself. So they said they really couldn't take him. He needs to be kept amused more, and he's going to day care. But now she has a heart condition and it's really getting to her. And she's just . . . one day it's fine and she doesn't think he needs to go, and the next day . . . you know. It's that back and forth. So she's going to try to get him into [another nursing home]."

Families may encounter waiting lists at good facilities and wrestle with financial arrangements while evaluating the relative merits of one home over another. Often local agencies on aging or the Alzheimer's Association can be of assistance. In addition to considering nursing home environment, quality of care, and types of services, families need to assess what staff members know about dementia and how they care for persons with dementing illnesses. Even though 60–80% of residents in nursing homes have some form of dementia (Rabins et al., 1999), institutional abilities to address their unique needs vary. First, resources differ in terms of nature and variety of opportunities for specialized programming and individualized attention. Second, general experience of staff working with people at various stages of dementia differ, often in relation to the educational and support resources available to them in their particular geographic area. Families need to educate themselves, tour resident areas, and ask about services, programming, and staff education that is targeted to dementia care.

Third, organizational approaches to care differ. Some homes integrate residents with cognitive impairment with residents who are cognitively intact. This can work well for certain individuals at particular stages of their illness. In addition, some homes have special care units (SCUs) that provide programs and activities tailored to interests and abilities of cognitively impaired people in an environment designed to meet their emotional and behavioral needs. These areas may provide safe havens for individuals whose acceptance in the general nursing home population is compromised by difficult to manage behaviors that are troubling to more cognitively intact residents and their families (e.g., rummaging, taking things, wandering, disrobing, and assaulting people). Then, there also are some nursing homes that try to simulate a family-style environment with small groupings of residents and staff who do natural everyday things together (e.g., folding laundry, baking cookies, potting plants) in more architecturally home-like settings. These arrangements strive to reproduce a familiar sense of belonging through positive social interaction in a relaxing atmosphere that may foster relationship formation and increase the functionality of some individuals. Beginning with the available options, families should expect discussion with nursing home personnel about the best person-environment fit. Lack of agreement between family and professional judgments on where the individual is most likely to function at his/her best in the nursing home environment sometimes occurs and will need to be resolved.

Facilities also vary in their philosophies about and abilities to accommodate aging in place (allowing residents to remain on the same unit throughout their nursing home course). Families may miss the significance of policies related to this because it seldom becomes an issue until later, when residents' further decline prompts discussions about moving them to other areas within the home. This helps facilities to group individuals by the level of care they require and free beds for other residents with special care needs.

A daughter explains: "I know that I signed it, and it's in the contract that 'We [the nursing home] can move people any time we want to' (worded much better than that, of course). But you're not reminded. And maybe you wouldn't want to be reminded all the time. So when things started to change [resident inactive and in need of total care] I was completely unprepared. I never entertained the idea that she'd be anywhere else. I have worried about [what would happen if she had to adjust to] a new aide. But [relocation was not a worry because] I thought this floor [special care unit] was her last move."

When making decisions about nursing home admission, families need to talk to staff and others with knowledge of the facility, make first-hand observations, and refer to reports related to the nursing home's licensure and inspection record. Different units and areas within a home will have their own environmental and social ambience. Therefore, ideas about the best in-house location for the individual also should be explored, with the understanding that what works well for any individual can change over time and usually is a matter of trial and error.

> A son recalls: "She just didn't fit the lifestyle on the [lower care level] floor, so they moved her. And that was really hard on me. I didn't like that at all because I liked the [other] floor better. It was quieter and the patients stayed to themselves. [Residents on the special care unit are more active.] And when they told me she was going to be moved, I didn't like it. But that was my problem. She is on the correct floor. I think that one of the reasons my mom was moved was because she was interfering with and bothering the other person in her room. She was annoying people . . . [taking their belongings]. [She thought] everything was hers."

Because the nursing home is a communal setting, persons with dementia may indeed have difficulty in recognizing boundaries between self and others and between the personal space and belongings of other residents and their own. In addition, the tolerance they may have encountered in home environments, where they might have been the sole focus of attention, changes. Thus, dealing with others' reactions and concerns is part of the adjustment that newly admitted residents and their families must make.

> For example, a wife expresses dismay over responses to her husband's confusion: "This floor [special care unit] is not as nice as the [other] floor. It doesn't bother my husband. It bothers me. [On the other floor] they said he was trying to get out the door, and when [the aide] tried to turn him around she said he tried to hit her. But that was the only incident. I think she exaggerated everything. And I know he wandered into some woman's room, and she got very upset. [Well,] for Pete's sake! The man doesn't know what he's doing."

Family members may have persistent concerns about in-house location of persons with dementia. These can arise from unavoidable comparisons with other residents. Symptoms of dementia will vary widely. Thus, family members may worry that the person will be disadvantaged by being with residents whose conditions, they believe, are more advanced. Feelings that their loved one is less afflicted than others, in turn, can feed upon and exacerbate insecurity or guilt that they might have experienced as a result of needing to admit the person to a nursing home.

A daughter explains why she believes that her mother should not be on the special care unit: "They took her cane away because of an incident with this woman who was constantly calling out for her husband. This annoyed my mother, and they got into a little tiffle. Now they claim my mother used her cane on this woman, [who then] bit my mother's hand. And then I said, 'You know, the confrontations would not be necessary if she were with people like herself.' So they tried her on another floor; but it was no better. [And I'm thinking] 'What did I do? What did I do [by admitting her]?' But my daughter said, 'You and Dad can't take care of Nana anymore!' And then my husband said, 'I think you're doing her an injustice if you let her think you'll take her out of here [as a result of these incidents]. This is where she belongs.' But, my mother isn't like [the other residents]. She doesn't look or act like she's lost her mind."

"I HAVE TO BE HER ADVOCATE."

Advocacy in the nursing home setting is an important but difficult role for family members. One way in which it can be difficult is in the challenge of balancing concerns about residents' needs against family members' needs to deal with the impact of the person's illness on their own lives. Thus, although resident and family member needs may be distinct, they often are inseparably intertwined. For instance, relocation issues that occur later in residents' stays, as previously noted, often involve moving from a more active unit to one with a resident mix that includes persons approaching the end of their lives. Persons in the last and most severe stages of dementia lose the ability to walk or sit without assistance, become less responsive, and are totally dependent in all aspects of care. The nursing home perspective may be that their places on special care units are needed for other residents who will receive benefits from that environment that they can no longer utilize. These changes, in time, may be seen to operate in some residents' best interests (e.g., when a more restful setting brings relief from an atmosphere that demands too much of their diminishing capacities for active engagement). However, the practice of aging in place that allows residents to stay in the same environment with familiar caregivers is very appealing to families. They want to avoid loss of continuity and of established ties with staff, residents, and other families that would accompany this type of change. Moreover, there may be anxiety about what the move signifies, that is, approaching end stages of the disease. And since no one really is ready for a loved one's death, even when it is anticipated, they may fear that observed differences resulting from the move may accelerate the person's decline, increasing guilt because they would hold themselves accountable. The following example illustrates one family member's anguish.

> *Daughter: "My mother is disruptive in groups. At this stage [of her dementia], too much stimulation bothers her; [and] she's total care. I thought the stroke would have taken her; but it didn't. So now I think it's the way it's supposed to be. I think God's allowing her to stay here [on earth] because this floor is the right place for her to be. And I think that's why she wants to stay [alive]. If she was miserable here, the stroke might have taken her. She might have let go and let it take her. So I'm against the move because she has bonded with these people [special care unit staff]. And my concern is that they're taking her away from what has become her extended family. These are the people she knows; and I think that being with strangers might bother her. Sometimes I look at her and think, 'Is anything going to bother her?' But I'm afraid this would be another step down [cause further decline] for her. Whenever there's a trauma she takes a big step down. She might be just fine on another floor. But I have to be her advocate; and I have to assume the worst to have the best for her."*

Advocacy outside of one's sphere of influence also can be difficult. Families find that although nursing home admission may relieve them of many worries and burdens of direct care, the new environment challenges them with a system that they cannot wholly control or always understand. Therefore, they need to continually evaluate whether they should accept, question, or challenge differences in nursing home staff members' ways of doing things. In the following example, a family member describes how the situation makes her feel like a "passenger" in a vehicle that she has been more accustomed to driving. The need for coordinated approaches across multiple caregivers in the nursing home setting adds complexity to the already complex trial and error nature of dementia care. And, as this family member observes, desired outcomes of some care approaches cannot be guaranteed. For her, advocacy involves an assumption that there is some logic in how staff members approach care, rationalization about placing trust in their professional judgments, and acceptance of their plans and actions as an act of faith.

Daughter: "Everybody's been great, and I think the care is extremely good. It's just little things every once in awhile. I imagine any family would feel like I do. You want to make sure whatever's going on is the best and in their [residents'] best interests. But a lot of times you don't understand. It's kind of like when you're a passenger in a car and you're always putting your foot on the [imaginary] brake. It's that kind of thing. [The staff] have got their procedures [ways of doing things]. They know where they're going, but you come into the middle of it, and you don't know that they have all these steps [plan of care]and that's where they're heading. You can say, 'Well, they're not there [desired outcome] yet.' But, you don't know that's where they're going to end up. They're very nice; but they can't guarantee it. There are times that I just have to trust that they'll do a good job."

Finally, in their advocate role, families must learn to be skilled interpreters of resident reports about what occurs in their absence. Because the resident with dementia cannot always construct a complete picture of what is going on, families must examine the evidence, observe and ask questions, and reflect on what meaning reported incidents and everyday happenings may hold for the person. The following is an example.

Daughter: "I know he has been violent. When he was at [the assisted living facility] he would tell me how people were coming in his windows and fighting with him. I'm not sure. I mean, I never saw any marks on him or anything there. Then when he got to [another facility], he again told me that people were beating him up. By then it became evident to me that he was the one . . . that when anybody would try to help him do anything (and he does need help), he would thrash out at them. Maybe somebody did try to restrain him. I don't really know. I don't know what I would do in that predicament either. [In this facility], about three or four weeks ago, he wanted to show me his hip where he got beat up. Well, when I asked, they showed me how they document everything and how a couple of days before [his report], he had fallen. He does fall. He has taken some good spills. [This time] he had become very violent when some aide had tried to help him. That was out in the hall [in view of others]. So, he was blaming them."

Evidence of injury and/or resident reports of mistreatment are serious matters that demand close investigation. If the resident has been deliberately hurt in some way by another, action will need to be taken to report and prevent further abuse. If the conclusion is that the resident's

account leaves out some critical details, it will be important to reinter-
pret the incident from his/her point of view. For instance, approaches
may need to be found that are less likely to result in the resident's
perception of care attempts as an assault. The question of whether
there had been an attempt in the past to restrain this resident is significant, since restraint can cause harm and, rather than decrease, often
will increase agitation. The daughter's reflection that she does not know
what she would do in such a predicament indicates empathy as well as
concern. As her father's advocate, she appropriately has tried to imagine
herself in his place, listened to him, and satisfied the need for more
information in pursuing his complaint.

Although some family members have deep feelings about their advocacy responsibilities, no family should feel that they are alone in this
role. Nursing home staff, across departments, often share similar feelings about being resident advocates in a system whose intricacies they
know well. Therefore, those who have been identified as the resident's
key care providers should be the first point of contact for questions
and concerns about care and services. They also can provide copies of
the Residents' Bill of Rights and interpret how it applies to given concerns. Families need to exercise their right to participate in care planning meetings and to insist on an opportunity to reschedule meeting
times that preclude their attendance. Regular meetings between family
members and staff provide opportunities for families to make suggestions, resolve conflict and communication problems, and establish their
roles as members of the interdisciplinary team responsible for providing
care to nursing home residents (Pillemer, Hegeman, Albright, & Henderson, 1998; Ryan & Scullion, 2000; Tickle & Hull, 1995).

If usual communication channels fail to produce satisfaction, families
may be able to receive support from community-based ombudsman/
adult protective services, whose role is to investigate unresolved issues,
provide mediation, make recommendations, and report evidence of
mistreatment. "The ombudsman program is authorized in the Older
Americans Act and administered by the Administration on Aging primarily through state and local area agencies on aging. Each state's
mandated ombudsman is expected to (1) investigate complaints made
by or on behalf of nursing home residents; (2) monitor the development
of federal, state, and local laws and regulations related to long-term
care; (3) provide information to families, agencies, policy makers and
other interested parties; and (4) coordinate training for staff and volunteers in each area agency . . . Local ombudsman programs typically seek
staff and volunteers motivated to serve institutionalized elderly in several

roles, including advocate, educator, investigator, observer, conflict me-diator, and friendly visitor" (Mason, 1995).

"I WANT TO GO HOME."

In the community, the sanctity of the "home" is upheld by social norms that encourage respect for individual privacy and personal property. Thus, people find sanctuary in their homes and experience a sense of violation when home boundaries are breached, as in the case of criminal trespass. In nursing homes, staff members often say, "This is the resi-dents' home" to convey the idea that similar principles should apply to the living circumstances of institutionalized elders. But many persons with dementia will not be able to understand why they are being thrust into a new environment and why someone does not take them "home." In the following example, a daughter suggests what some residents' pleas to be rescued from the situation might signify.

> "It's heartbreaking to have to listen to, 'I want to go home, I want to go home; take me home, I want to go home.' And so many people [families] are just torn by that. But, you know, they [residents] don't really want to go to a place. They want to go to the way life was before, and it's not something you can do. And even if you took them home . . . I took my mother home many times and she still wasn't happy. She wanted life to be the way it was before, and that just can't be. This [perspective] could ease some families' guilt."

Although this is one possible interpretation of what wanting to go home could mean to residents, it is not the only possibility. Wanting to go home also might be a response to what the experience of being in a nursing home is like. Most people would not choose to live in a nursing home if there were ways to avoid it. Nursing home residents are separated from the rest of society. Their daily lives are organized around imposed routines that make it possible to care for them as a group (or in small groups). Most are strangers to one another when they first arrive, yet everyone lives in close proximity, sharing sleeping quarters, bathrooms, dining facilities, lounges, and other public areas. Thus, numerous studies of nursing home culture portray it as lacking in homelike qualities, threatening to personal identity, and demoraliz-ing to the human spirit.

Gubrium (1975), in his description of *Living and Dying in Murray Manor,* used the phrase "bed and body work" to discuss depersonalization (loss of individuality) of residents by staff members' task-oriented imposition of daily routines designed to meet institutional requirements for maximum efficiency in meeting their most visible needs. As a consequence, individual choices and preferences were disregarded and consideration of residents' less visible human needs (social, emotional, and spiritual) was subordinated to an emphasis on custodial care.

In her comparison of nursing home life in the United States and Scotland, Kayser-Jones (1981) also observed depersonalizing regimentation governing group treatment of residents. Her study described a greater tendency toward this in the United States. She extensively analyzed and discussed nursing home practices resulting in depersonalization (loss of individuality) and other principal problems of nursing home life, identified as infantilization (treating older people like children), dehumanization (loss of dignity and sense of self-worth), and victimization (inflicting harm through specific acts, such as theft or abuse, or the overall psychological harm of depersonalization, infantilization, and dehumanization). Kayser-Jones theorized that the power-dependence ratio in nursing homes (residents being dependent and staff having the power) provides insight into these problems. She observed that—"In power-dependence relations, individuals who need services have the following options: (1) they can supply a service in return, (2) they may obtain the service elsewhere, (3) they can use coercion to obtain the service, (4) they may choose to do without the service. If they are unable to choose any of these alternatives, they must comply with the wishes of the one in power since he can make the continuing supply of the needed service contingent upon compliance" (p. 113).

Although power balances may be encountered at home, at work, at school, and in other areas of life, the isolation and dependency of nursing home residents makes them more vulnerable than adults in other settings. Therefore, it should not be assumed that compliant residents who seldom complain are content with their circumstances. Families and nursing home staff need to be aware of the environmental factors that influence residents' repression of unexpressed wishes and concerns. There are additional factors to consider if the resident's dementia causes him/her to be anxious, suspicious, or paranoid, as the following conversations with a resident and her daughter illustrate.

CARE CONCERNS—"THAT'S NOT MY IDEA . . . BUT I WOULD NEVER SAY ANYTHING."

Resident: "I eat breakfast in the dining room most of the time. I get up early [in order to get to the dining room], but I don't mind [because]I don't like to eat in my room. I don't like to eat in bed. [Bedtime] is too early, though . . . about seven thirty or eight o'clock. That's not my idea. They put me to bed when they want to, but I would never say anything."

Researcher: "Why not? Couldn't you say you'd like to stay up longer?"

Resident: "Oh, I would never . . . ! Now I'm worried. I don't want you to tell. That would be just awful if you told."

Daughter: "At least you can watch TV in bed, Mother."

Resident: "No, they don't let me watch TV. I would like to watch TV, but they turn it off."

Daughter: "Why? Is it because your roommate is sleeping?"

Resident: "Oh, I don't know. She sleeps all the time. Now I don't want you reporting this because it would cause an awful lot of trouble if anyone found out I said something. Oh dear, oh dear, oh dear!" [Daughter resolves to follow up.]

Staffing patterns, the number of residents assigned to an individual caregiver, and those residents' needs and levels of functional independence will determine when individuals who need assistance will get out of bed in the morning, be taken to the toilet, bathe, dress, eat, and go to bed at night. This extreme dependence on the availability of helpers for the most basic human requirements and the subordination of personal needs to workers' job demands and schedules is the norm for nursing home residents. In this example, when the meal trays arrive, the need for staff to serve and assist residents with breakfast will curtail morning care for awhile. Therefore, residents who are not ready to go to the dining room will be served in their rooms. This resident's acceptance of rising early in the morning enables her to eat breakfast where she wishes—in the dining room, not in her bed. However, she reports that her too early bedtime routine does not offer a similar quid pro quo, since even watching television is not an option. Details are not forthcoming in response to listeners' questions because the focus rapidly shifts to the resident's anxious pleas that they treat the information as a confidence that, if divulged, would place her in jeopardy.

The resident's reluctance to communicate her preference may illustrate powerlessness experienced by individuals whose basic daily activities are scheduled and controlled by other people. Fear of retribution as punishment for complaining always must be seen as a possibility. However, fear need not be based on objective reality. Rather, dependence on the benevolence of care providers who have the power to give or to withhold is a sufficient psychological threat to make anything short of acquiescence seem ungrateful (evidence of dehumanization/

loss of self-worth) as well as too risky to contemplate (victimization/ fear of harm). Follow-up of the resident's concerns will need to be accomplished in a protective and careful manner.

An important consideration in this case is that the resident's fear of negative consequences, if her complaint is made known, also may be related to her dementia.

> *Daughter: "She's been really paranoid about a lot of things. And they started her on a different medication because she was so anxious. Of course she thought they were giving her something that was bad for her. She insisted I take Dad's picture home because she didn't know what they would do with it; and she didn't want him to be implicated in anything. She thought she was on a list, that people were saying she was dishonest and everybody was talking about her, that they thought she was a nuisance and they got her roommate believing it. [When we talk,] she'll say, 'Now, shut the door. I don't want anybody to hear.' This went on all week. So I asked the doctor to take her off that medicine. She was so paranoid, I couldn't stand it. So it was stopped, and she seemed real good (not paranoid anymore). But she was just [very anxiously repeating]—'Oh dear, oh dear, oh dear' and always worried about something. In fact, one day, one of the aides called me and asked, 'Would you just talk to your mother? She thinks you've been in an accident.' So it's obvious, I guess, that she does need something to calm her down. But they've got to find the right medication. They're going to try something new, and I'll be anxious to see how she is with it."*

Some persons with dementia develop false ideas about the meaning of what is going on around them based on misinterpretations of what others do and say. Difficulty in remembering what they are told combined with inability to interpret others' actions, questions, directions, or explanations may lead to suspiciousness and paranoia. This could be seen as a natural consequence of being held captive by an injured mind in a world that increasingly makes no sense. In an effort to make sense of the world around them, individuals may conclude that they are in danger from others who intend to do them harm. Discovery of the right medication (dependent on individual tolerances) may provide relief from troubling psychological symptoms. In addition, it is important to evaluate vision and hearing because persons with dementia may not be aware of sensory deficits that impede interpretation of environmental cues. However, if it is the brain that misinterprets what the eyes and ears see and hear clearly, persons will need frequent, patient, nonconfrontational repetition of accurate information about the sights, sounds, and actions taking place around them.

Worry, anxiety, agitation, and restlessness are other symptoms that some persons with dementia experience. Sometimes these symptoms may be a direct result of the brain disease, but possible medical causes, such as undiagnosed pain, will need to be ruled out. Symptoms could be a response to individuals not knowing where they are or what is expected of them. Or persons could be depressed over multiple losses, including loss of a sense of control over their lives from being able to carry out their own routines in a more familiar environment. Environments and/or care providers that exert control over all aspects of a person's life also can produce these kinds of reactions.

In summary, there are multiple factors that can contribute to the distress of nursing home residents with dementia. Some involve reactions to loss, unfamiliarity of surroundings, or rhythms of nursing home life and/or actions of care providers that contribute to depersonalization and dehumanization. Some involve changing medical status, which bears close monitoring since residents may be limited in their abilities to report medical symptoms. And some involve ongoing pathological changes affecting cognition, behavior, and personality that are beyond anyone's control. In the following examples, families mourn and describe the effects of these disease-related losses.

Daughter: "It's so important to understand that this person really isn't the person he was to begin with—that we knew when we were younger. Otherwise you just get so upset. You walk out after a visit [feeling so] empty, [thinking], 'This is life!' . . . And, being a family member, I always worry about myself. You know—What's in store for me?"

Daughter: "I don't really think of this person as my mother. I call her Mom, but I don't think of her as my mother. My mother is gone. I visit this person because if there is anything of my mother left, I love that part. . . . And, I hope that somehow she knows that we haven't deserted her."

Son: "You wonder, does she think? Does she have thoughts in her head that she can't get out? It's like watching your mother die slowly as opposed to, you know, [the suddenness of] getting a phone call that she's passed away. It's just a constant [source of sorrow]."

Because the causes of residents' distress may come simultaneously from many directions, considering all the possibilities is essential. For instance, neither the nature of nursing home life nor the destructive effect of dementia on intellect and personality may be solely accountable for the variety of worries and upsets that residents may experience. But both may take their toll. Therefore, cognitively impaired residents, especially residents whose disease symptoms include suspiciousness or paranoia, always must be taken seriously because the possibility that they are responding to restrictions, depersonalization, or actual threats in their environment cannot be discounted. Failure to accept that their signs of distress or voiced concerns may be based on such reality is dehumanizing and places them at risk of being victimized. All behavior has meaning. What residents with dementia need from others is a respectful person-centered attitude consistent with Kitwood's (1998) "ethic of context." Being attentive to each individual's unique experience and life history is at the heart of this ethic, which involves "engag[ing] with the context [the flow of everyday life that envelops the person with dementia] as well as the issues" (p. 24) and "look[ing] for possible meaning in [every] action and utterance, even when it appears to be bizarre, incoherent, or disgusting" (p. 27).

SOCIAL CONCERNS—"DAYS ARE SLOW AND NOT VERY INTERESTING."

Calendars of organized activities for nursing home residents typically list a variety of opportunities for active participation (e.g., singing, crafts, games, trips, parties, exercise and interest groups) and spectator entertainment (e.g., movies, performances). Generally, these activities are the responsibility of on-staff recreation therapists, although volunteers play a significant role in some facilities. Pastoral care staff or area clergy also may assume responsibility for conducting worship services and organizing spiritual care activities. Residents with dementia are included in large group activities if they are willing to go and are not too disruptive. However, small groups often are better for meeting their special needs, and some persons benefit most from one-to-one contact. Some facilities are able to assign staff to a particular unit in order to focus more on these small group and individual social and recreational needs. This creates more possibilities for tailoring activities to residents' interests and abilities.

Residents' engagement with daily activities depends on discovering what is meaningful to them. Learning about residents' habits, interests, and desires is better accomplished by spending time with and learning more about them as individuals than by relying on simply asking them if they would like to participate in a planned activity. Residents with dementia may not understand the invitation or what it involves. Some may automatically say "no" even when they really might mean "yes." Some might enjoy the activity but may not wish to leave the perceived safety of the unit or attend off-unit events unaccompanied by a familiar person. It also is possible that available activities do not fit a resident's present needs. Encouraging continuity with past interests is an optimal goal. Persons who can no longer master a skill they once enjoyed (e.g., sewing, painting, or carpentry) also may find comfort in reminiscing about or handling materials and tools involved in these pastimes. Conversely, past pleasures may frustrate or no longer hold the person's interest. Thus, new activities will need to match current abilities and tolerances. Many residents with dementia can clearly state their preferences and choose whether or not to participate in available offerings. They need to have control over these decisions. Observing the nonverbal behavior of residents who cannot express themselves in words or who have grown listless and apathetic is important. Simply positioning them to receive positive feedback from whatever is going on in the environment (e.g., human touch, presence and interaction; pleasing sensations, sights, sounds, and smells) may provide clues—facial expressions, utterances, gestures, and subtle body language. Sensitivity to how individuals respond to activity taking place around them also will reveal which persons benefit from increased social stimulation and which individuals need quieter, less distracting surroundings.

The issue of discovering what is meaningful to people was a central concern of Savishinsky's (1991) study of life and work in a nursing home. The following was an important finding: "Recreation programs had unintended consequences and meanings for residents. The pet therapy sessions, for example, were designed primarily to provide elderly [residents] with an hour or two of animal contact each week. But for many individuals, the social and sensory stimulation of the pets was superceded in importance by the interpersonal ties with the volunteers who brought them. Human rather than animal companionship thus became the most rewarding experience for many" (p. 240).

It follows from this understanding that planned group activities, although more efficient and economical from the facility's point of view, will not satisfy individual needs for more naturally occurring personal human contact. Additionally, Savishinsky's work illustrated residents' needs for more than just companionship: "[T]hey wanted communication . . . they desired to be seen, spoken to, heard, and held" (p. 241). He reported that caregivers and volunteers found residents with dementia to be the most challenging in this regard because of their unpre-

dictability, distractibility, language/communication difficulties, and si-
lences. Success in relating and responding to them was linked to individual tolerances. For instance, use of touch and sharing company in
silence was comforting to some, but not all, residents. "Nor were all
staff and volunteers equally comfortable with touch and silence as means
of communication" (p. 242).

Residents need human relationships and they also need a sense of
personal autonomy. They may socialize and participate in organized
activities yet, nevertheless, feel that these distractions do not compensate
for lost independence in directing particular daily routines that used
to make life meaningful. For example, the following conversation was
in response to the question, "What do you do all day?"

*Resident: "I watch people [and] we just sit around and talk. Days are
slow and not very interesting."*

*Daughter: "When she was home, she had her tasks to do, whether it was
dishes, or mopping the floor, or laundry on certain days. And that's gone.
So I think that [contributes to] the idea that there's nothing to do even
though there's all these activities going on, and she's participating. It's
not her routine. There's this setup now [the nursing home's routine] where
[everything] is done for her."*

The loss of personal autonomy experienced by this resident resulted
in a diminished interest and sense of engagement in life. Her routines
at home had a purpose that is lacking in the nursing home, where
everything is done for her. Savishinsky (1991) observed that some residents who miss a former lifestyle respond to institutional regimes by
creating their own routines built around some meaningful activity. He
also noted that "the apparently passive pursuit of watching" was found
to be a meaningful, engaging activity for some residents (p.119). The
resident in the example provides some evidence of this. However, her
daughter worries that her use of lifelong skills to adapt socially to those
around her will be a disadvantage if she is among others who cannot
communicate. Consequently, her concerns about the resident's in-
house placement turn on this issue.

Researcher: "What kinds of things do you like to do?"
Resident: "Nothing. I don't like to do anything."
Researcher: "You said that you watch people."
Resident: "Yes. I do like that. They don't know it."

Researcher: "They don't know you're watching?"

Resident: "That's right. Yes, I like that."

Daughter [in a later conversation]: "She's always been a very social person. . . . She's kind of a chameleon and will adapt to her surroundings. [If people talk to her] she brightens up. But [with] people she can't talk to, or that won't talk to her, she will withdraw . . . [And] she's very perceptive. She notices little things that you just don't always expect . . . [On the special care unit] she pretty much stayed in her room [and] hid out. She knew those people [residents] wouldn't talk to her. And it was traumatic for me. We knew that [if she remained there] it would be the end. [After she was moved to another unit] I came in and she was playing games. She's got a wonderful roommate, and she's integrating more."

Creating community in institutional settings often does involve moving, grouping, and regrouping residents in hopes of finding "good matches" of individual personalities. And confronting boredom and loss of purpose in days that are perceived by residents as "slow and not too interesting" poses challenges in a communal environment where there is diversity in individual interests, habits, and abilities. Some residents say they are bored; others say they are not. Some residents form new friendships and become socially active. (One daughter said about her mother: "She worked hard all her life [and] this is the first social life she's had.") Yet other residents withdraw. Some residents say, "I've always been a loner." Other residents come into their element as activists and leaders. Responses to opportunities for social engagement may be mediated by fatigue or discomfort from illness and physical/cognitive incapacity that affect residents' levels of participation and how they perceive the quality of their lives. Diversity of the population may not be the only issue, however. Nursing homes differ in the quality, extent, and appropriateness of daily life amenities and leisure time opportunities that are available to residents.

ENVIRONMENTAL CONCERNS—"SHARING A ROOM WAS VERY HARD."

Daughter: "She had [several different] roommates. Some she got along with; and some [did not work out]very well. We didn't blame it on the roommate, especially. I mean, it was maybe half and half. But it was the sharing of a room. [Sharing a room] was very hard, and I can understand that."

Wife: "He kept [his roommate—"R"] up at night [wandering and rummaging]. It wasn't good [between the two of them]. He started to wander over onto ["R's"] side of the room. And ["R"] would kinda grab him by the arm and say, 'No! Go back!' or something. And [my husband] told me that he was very rude. But that wasn't so. That was just his interpretation."

Daughter: "This woman that shares the room thinks that my mother is her mother.And she hovers over her . . . and gets in her bed just to be close to her. She must be [hanging] on her constantly, the poor soul. [But] it's frustrating to my mother."

The restrictive nature of nursing home settings places a premium on a person's enjoyment of life. Nursing home residents often experience frustration, loneliness, and boredom in sterile institutional settings where they endure crowding, sharing room and bath facilities with strangers, engaging in close daily contact with persons whose behavior is unfriendly and disturbing, and waiting indefinitely, it seems, for staff to attend to their personal needs. Residents tend to see themselves as having little in common with one another. And, to some extent, the heterogeneity of the population bears this out. It also is difficult for nursing homes, which increasingly are expected to be "all things to all people," to satisfy everyone all the time. The following background understandings suggest past and current considerations that contextualize some of these environmental concerns.

PROVIDING MANY DIFFERENT THINGS TO MANY DIFFERENT PEOPLE

There is a kind of uniformity in perceptions of nursing homes as long-term care facilities for the elderly that understates their current heterogeneous nature. Nursing homes offer a wide breadth of programs and services. They may be closely or loosely affiliated with hospital systems and many provide beds for patients of all ages who are in convalescence post-surgery or receiving rehabilitation following strokes, fractures, and other injuries. For these individuals, length of stay usually is short, consistent with the goal of returning them to the community. Short-term stays at the other end of the care continuum include terminally ill individuals who can no longer be maintained at home or at lower-level care facilities and often die in less than a year. These persons have complex medical needs and require skilled professional care to assure physical comfort and psychosocial support. Nursing homes also admit comatose individuals who need continuous and sometimes highly technical care for undetermined lengths of time. And many nursing homes also have day and respite programs that provide personal care and socialization to community-based elders and support to their caregivers.

In contrast, long-term-stay residents include alert and cognitively intact individuals, the majority of whom are elderly, whose chronic illnesses and physical disabilities require them to live in a protective environment where personal care and assistance with daily living are available. However, residents at different stages of dementia also make up a large and growing proportion of the long-term stay nursing home population. All long-term residents need an environment that can support their everyday needs for maintaining normalcy of lifestyle, autonomy, dignity, and privacy. For cognitively intact persons, this also includes encouraging their cooperation and understanding of other residents' needs and limitations, but not forcing residents with dementia upon them. Persons with dementia require care that is tailored to their unique needs in a supportive environment that is capable of maximizing their remaining abilities to function personally and socially.

Clearly, nursing homes are expected to be many things to many people—people with vastly different individual characteristics and capacities, immediate needs, and future expectations who are admitted for different reasons and stay for varied lengths of time. On the one hand, as residences, they are expected to provide a homelike social environment that is conducive to persons' emotional, psychological, and spiritual well-being. On the other hand, as health care facilities, they must be able to monitor and treat medically complex physical conditions of residents that, at times, develop into needs for emergency and acute care services. Nursing home caregivers have to attend to some acute care needs and sometimes arrange short-term transfers of residents to hospital settings for medically stabilizing treatment. However, adjusting to differences between nursing home and hospital cultures can be traumatic for persons in these circumstances.

Nursing homes may be large or small; public, for-profit, or not-for-profit; and more or less homogeneous in resident and staff population. They are different in terms of setting and location within the community; architectural and organizational structure; and variety of institutional resources, services, and amenities. Each facility has its own culture as well as multiple subcultures that make up the whole. When nursing home culture is spoken of in the abstract, it represents the more general historical and collective experience of these types of institutions. But, broadly speaking, nursing home culture, as discussed in the literature, cannot be understood apart from the larger social and political systems within which it exists. The human and social diversity within these facilities has led them to be described as cultural microcosms of society. Yet, it is a society from which they often are curiously isolated and estranged.

HISTORICAL BACKGROUND

Over the years, nursing homes have occupied an ambiguous position in American society, charged with charitably meeting human needs for shelter and assistance while operationally exacting what has been perceived as a great price in terms of human dignity and freedom. Some homes trace their origins to old age homes of 150 or more years ago that were founded by religious congregations or benevolent societies. Other facilities were founded as county almshouses for the poor. The original emphasis on community-based support in providing food and shelter for the frail, disabled, orphaned, and elderly had less of the medical focus of contemporary nursing homes. However, in the 1950s, recognition of a need for better health care for a growing aged segment of the population encouraged government lending policies that favored changes in more modest existing homes for the aged and construction of new nursing homes that were more hospital-like in appearance and function (R. A. Kane, R. L. Kane, & Ladd, 1998). The 1965 passage of Medicare and Medicaid legislation further fueled expansion of the nursing home industry. But with it came rising incidents of insufficient oversight. Care of persons in nursing homes suffered as attention focused on an evolving real estate market and the ownership and management of homes changed hands. Publications chronicling poor conditions, neglect, and abuse of nursing home residents began to appear with titles such as: *Too Old, Too Sick, Too Bad: Nursing Homes in America* (Moss & Halamandaris, 1977) or *Why Survive? Being Old in America* (Butler, 1968). The scandals of this period led to a review of nursing home standards in the 1980s and passage of legislation known as OBRA '87 (Omnibus Budget Reconciliation Act of 1987). Consequently, nursing home regulations were strengthened, with an emphasis being placed on quality of life (e.g., dignity, privacy, relationship formation, and social participation); residents' rights; training of nursing assistants; and a mandated inspection process. Regular inspections now were to include obtaining direct information from residents about their care as well as observing their actual conditions, especially with an eye toward reducing the overall use of physical and chemical restraints (R. A. Kane et al., 1998). Nevertheless, societal fears about inadequate, abusive care and disenchantment with nursing homes as places in which to live constitute a current and ongoing theme.

In the 1970s and '80s, anthropologists began to examine everyday life in nursing homes using the same techniques employed by this discipline to study small bounded societies (Gubrium, 1975; Henderson, 1981, 1987; Kayser-Jones, 1981; O'Brien, 1989; Powers, 1988a, 1988b; Shield, 1988; Vesperi, 1983, 1995; Watson & Maxwell, 1977). This involved spending time in one or a small number of homes and informally observing, talking, and interacting with individuals in their usual rounds of daily activities (participant observation); identifying issues and points of interest; and conducting in-depth interviews. The resulting cultural portraits of nursing home worlds combined subjective perspectives of their inhabitants (the insider point of view) and analytical interpretations of what meanings or understandings might be derived from appreciation of those perspectives (the scientist's rendering of revealed cultural realities). In many ways these studies confirmed and presented in greater detail the difficult challenges to residents and staff of living and working in nursing homes. But they also brought forward a more complicated picture of human experience in these facilities, illustrating how the cultural landscape looks different through the eyes of individuals at varying places in the social and organizational structure. In his introduction to Henderson and Vesperi's (1995) collection of ethnographers' contributions to the field of gerontology, Stafford (1995) comments on the effect and the purpose of applying an anthropological lens to the multiple perspectives that surface through these studies.

> Readers will find that there are no clear 'good guys' or 'bad guys' in a nursing home. The actors operate on the basis of their perspectives and while we should be aware of the consequences of perspectives, those who hold them often do so for benevolent, or at least benign, reasons . . . Still ethnography itself does not promote social action. What it does promote, when done well, is understanding, and understanding leads to respect for all the players in this human drama. (p. x)

Respect as an outcome of understanding others' points of view is an important aspect of ethical action. For example, reports that pay attention to how nursing home residents and staff feel about themselves, their circumstances, and how others treat them often speak about ways in which living and working in these settings is associated with various forms of stigmatization. On the one hand, residents are faced with the stigma of being old, sick, and shut away from the world—placed in a category with other people whose varied and questionable conditions threaten an already weakened sense of self-worth. Especially questionable are the conditions of persons with dementia, from whose presence other residents most often attempt to distance themselves (Goffman, 1961; Gubrium, 1975; Savishinsky, 1991; Shield, 1988). On the other hand, staff are faced with the stigma of society's negative image of nursing home employment and lack of appreciation of the caregiving challenges in these settings (Foner, 1994a, 1994b; Reinhard, Barber, Mezey, Mitty, & Peed, 2002). Failure to understand how social and cultural attitudes influence daily life in institutions promotes criticism and confrontation. However, Savishinsky (1991) observes that "when greater understanding is achieved about stigmatized individuals, the result is generally a more humane consideration of their human needs and civil rights" (p. 142).

FINDING ONE'S SPOT

> *Researcher: "What do you do all day?"*
>
> *Resident: "We eat. That's what we do. I have my place in the dining room. They like to put you in a certain spot, and that's your place."*
>
> *Researcher: "Tell me about your place."*
>
> *Resident: "Oh, it's all right. [I eat with] the same woman. The food is good, and they let you change it [menu items] if you want to."*
>
> *Wife: "That's his spot [in the dining room/day room]. When he was still walking, he used to automatically go over to that area so [now that he is chair-bound]I just appropriated it because he can see the whole room and can connect. And do you know [that other residents also claim space]? One of my grandchildren was sitting in that chair one day, and T.R. came in and said [in an anxious voice], 'Where do I go? Where do I go? Where do I go?' And I said, 'I think you're sitting in her chair. So she got up, and then T.R. sat right down."*

The above quotations provide a literal translation of what it can mean to "find one's spot" in a nursing home environment. They illustrate tendencies on the part of staff to "place" people as well as residents' needs to claim space for themselves. But, in a larger sense, finding one's spot also may signify attaining recognition as an individual through formation of personal relationships with others in the nursing home community.

A current emphasis on nursing home culture change supports this important human need. Culture change is a social movement that aims at empowering residents and staff to create more comfortable homelike environments that are energized by and grounded in positive and respectful human relationships. Historically, a variety of streams of work and thought have contributed to this effort.

First, systematic study and advocacy to reduce the use of physical and chemical restraints in nursing homes has focused on observed dangers and negative effects such as serious injuries, deaths, increased agitation, regression, depression, and demoralization (Capezuti, Strumpf, Evans, Grisso, & Maislin, 1998; Castle, Fogel, & Mor, 1997; Castle & Fogel, 1998; Dunbar, Neufeld, White, & Libow, 1996; Miles & Irving, 1992; C. C. Williams & Finch, 1997). Advocating for restraint-free nursing homes was an early rallying point for new standards of care that consider the well-being of the whole person—physically (i.e., preventing harm) and socially (i.e., restoring human rights, a sense of control, respect and dignity) (Evans & Strumpf, 1989; R. L. Kane, C. C. Williams, T. F. Williams, & R. A. Kane, 1993; Moss & La Puma, 1991; C. C. Williams, 1989).

Second, literature on individualized care systematically has stressed putting the person before the routine or procedure by trying to understand the situation from his/her perspective (Beck, Heacock, Rapp, & Mercer, 1993; Happ, C. C. Williams, Strumpf, & Burger, 1996; Rader, 1994, 1995; Rader, Lavelle, Hoeffer, & McKenzie, 1996; Vogelpohl, Beck, Heacock, & Mercer, 1996). Consequently, recommended strategies for meeting care needs of persons with dementia, such as bathing and other activities of daily living, are based on using specific knowledge about individuals (e.g., past patterns and current preferences) to develop approaches that are tailored to their wishes, abilities, limitations, and tolerances.

Third, strategies for changing the social and organizational climates of nursing homes have been described and demonstrated. Some of these approaches have involved environmental modifications to create smaller, more intimate groupings of residents (e.g., "neighborhoods") as well as cross-training of staff and decentralization of departments into smaller multifunctional teams that provide direct service to residents (Boyd, 1994). The Regenerative Community Model developed at one home uses daily community meetings to communicate values of the culture, that is, that there remains in each person, regardless of infirmity, "a part . . . that is still healthy and capable of learning, growth, and renewal" (Barkan, 1995, p. 172). Through a community development process, residents sing, exercise, talk, plan activities, and engage in celebrations and rituals designed to give each a voice and a sense of connection.

The Eden Alternative (Thomas, 1994, 1996, 1999) probably has received the most widespread recognition. It focuses on creating human habitats that enable residents to grow, thrive, and enjoy meaningful connections with people associated with the facility (e.g., each other, caregivers, families, volunteers, children in on-site or special day care programs) as well as people in the community at large (e.g., participation in public affairs or political action groups and committees; membership in clubs related to hobbies and special interests). This human habitat model seeks to encourage relationship formation and enhancement of inter-personal interaction by simultaneously transforming physical environments and organizational structures. Transformation of physical environments involves introducing homelike comforts that are aesthetically pleasing, stimulate interest, and encourage relaxation (e.g., architectural and interior design modifications of institutional facilities; multisensory interventions such as music, aromatherapy, special use of color, light, sounds and textures; natural surroundings—plants, flowers, gardens, water effects; and introduction of biologic diversity in the form of multispecies resident companions such as dogs, cats, rabbits, hamsters, birds, and fish). Additionally, transformation of organizational structures involves change from a top-down administrative model to a decentralized team model where staff members are empowered to manage themselves and their assignments. Upper level management acts in an advisory capacity to multidisciplinary teams and committees that share responsibilities for the smooth operation of the facility and cooperate in identifying and addressing resident, family, and staff issues and concerns.

Since the original research that marked its inception, descriptive accounts of results of "Edenization" (or "the EA") in various facilities suggest that its endorsed changes in nursing home culture have a positive impact on residents' quality of life (Barba, Tesh, & Courts, 2002). However, the causal connections between improved quality of life and outcomes related to quality of care remain open to further study. For example, it has been claimed that fewer infections resulting in lower use of antibiotics and improved quality of life resulting in decreased use of psychotropic drugs translate into a variety of improvements in resident well-being and lower costs in specific EA homes (Thomas, 1994; Henkel, 2000). However, generalizability of these findings has not been established. A recent study of two homes operated by the same organization—an EA study site and a control—found "no beneficial effects of the EA in terms of cognition, functional status, survival, infection rate, or cost of care after 1 year" (Coleman et al., 2002, p. M422). At the same time, the anecdotal data showed that residents and staff perceived that quality of life changes effected by the EA were positive. These researchers concluded that determining the relationship between the EA and specified quality of care outcomes may take longer than one year. They also advise that future studies will need to control for other factors such as "burden of illness" (e.g., numbers of acutely and terminally ill residents) and take into consideration that staff turnover may increase during the first year of EA implementation. Their study illustrates a need to take apart and examine individually the relationships between quality of life EA variables and quality of care outcomes. The demographics of nursing home populations that, on a broad geographic scale vary widely, need to be considered as well. An EA goal is to "optimize medical treatment" by keeping it "in its proper place," as "servant of genuine human caring, never its master" (Thomas, 1999, p. 97, 144). Understanding what this interplay between the EA quality of life philosophy and clinical care/treatment looks like for different nursing home resident populations with different mixes of health care needs may clarify what the goals and expectations of nursing homes that undertake to put its principles into practice should be.

An unfortunate outgrowth of above described initiatives to improve nursing home life has been a tendency to pit the *quality of life* focus of "social models" (associated with resident autonomy by supporters) against the *quality of care* focus of "medical/health care models" (associated with resident dependency by critics). R. A. Kane et al. (1998) call these distinctions "dysfunctional," asserting that clinical ("therapeutic") care with its emphasis on physical and mental health and supportive ("compensatory") care with its emphasis on social and spiritual well-being are two related aspects of long-term care that are of equal importance. And they maintain that the operational definitions of *quality of care* and *quality of life* "have more in common than many people realize . . . [Therefore,] one must grapple with this duality and satisfy the requirements of each" (pp. 192, 195).

In this spirit and in consideration of the fact that nursing homes must care for an increasing number of seriously ill and debilitated older people, a registered nurse wrote the following:

> *"It seems to me, in long-term care, that we have lost something concerning nursing care of the resident. We are quick to look at nursing care and label it "The Medical Model" and want a more social plan of action. I see long-term care as having a dual challenge of providing quality nursing care and creating a homelike setting. . . . It is my belief that some of the difficulties we have with families and residents can be solved by providing quality nursing care rather than just social care. For difficult behaviors,*

a behavioral flow chart with planned interventions is not always tried,
for example. I believe families admit people to a nursing facility for care
by nurses. Quality nursing care is an important part of solutions."

Quality nursing care—regardless of a facility's organizational structure
(top-down or decentralized team)—directs, supports, and enhances the
efforts of nursing assistants, who constitute the industry's primary hands-
on care workforce. Harrington et al. (2000) cite many studies that
consistently show a relationship between higher ratios of registered
and licensed practical nurse hours and significant improvements in
residents' quality of care. In addition, Reinhard et al. (2002) suggest
that new/expanded roles of advanced practice nurses in nursing homes
may increase effectiveness of primary nursing staff in decreasing quality
of care deficiencies in state and federal surveys.

NURSING HOMES AND LONG TERM CARE— "IT'S THE WAY SOCIETY IS TODAY."

Grief and guilt associated with nursing home admission sometimes is
tinged with nostalgia for times when it is believed that there were fewer
obstacles to caring for family members in the community and less need
to resort to institutional services.

For example, a wife said: "It's the way society is today. I just thank God
for nursing homes because with the family unit the way it is—man and
woman working and then if they have a parent . . . they give up their job,
one of them . . . It's not like years ago [when] Grandma and Grandpa
moved in with the family to be taken care of. It isn't like that anymore."

However, advocates of long-term care reform suggest that institutionalization would not be a foregone conclusion if elders had more options
and if there was less reliance on informal care systems (i.e., family,
friends, and neighbors) to pick up the slack in the absence of adequate,
coordinated community based services. Nursing home care is very expensive and, in the United States, it receives the larger portion of public
(federal and state) funding. Nevertheless, despite a national bias toward
institutional care, there is a deep-seated belief within the general popu-
lace that people should be able to receive care in the least restrictive
environment. Nursing homes, as they currently exist, are the most
restrictive environments and represent the preferred choice of no one.

The presence of dementia adds to the difficulties of estimating risk-benefit ratios of community-based versus nursing home care in individual cases. Many cognitively impaired persons function adequately and more happily at home, living alone or with family members. There are some instances where nursing home admission is held at bay until there seems to be no other recourse, but there also are situations where persons seemingly are forced into nursing homes against their wishes because of others' worries about safety (Waymack, 2001). In the absence of clear danger, worries may be concretely linked to an insufficient community-based support system or they may be general and nonspecific. For instance, grief over a person's frailty and decline may lead to fear that surely some catastrophe is bound to happen if steps are not taken to avoid it. Since life anywhere can never be totally risk-free, the steps to be taken are not always clear. Institutionalization is a step that some take in hopes that persons will be safer, physically. However, individuals can be harmed in other ways. For example, persons with dementia who can function to some degree in a familiar setting but are less able to deal with the combined stress of diminishing abilities and confusing changes in their lives may be more frustrated and function less well in a nursing home environment. In fact, it has been suggested that keeping persons out of nursing homes longer through better subsidized comprehensive home services, family caregiver relief, and more suitable residential alternatives, might lower the incidence of anxious, aggressive behaviors on the part of individuals who come to these settings sooner than they might need to for lack of better alternatives (R. A. Kane et al., 1998). Overall, the combination of concerns about safety and a long-term care system that tilts toward nursing home care as the solution highlights difficult ethical issues that are complicated by imbalances of funding in the public service sphere. The ambivalence people feel about "tradeoffs" between their safety and their freedom (R. A. Kane & Levin, 2001; R. A. Kane et al., 1998) has been described as "the ethical tightrope we walk" (Dubler & Nimmons, 1992):

> How do we best empower and not abandon? How do we helpfully support an elderly person without imposing our own narrow vision of her safety and well-being? We do not want to force them to be something they are not, yet we still want to protect them from unknowingly injuring themselves or suffering needlessly. (p. 194)

For many individuals, the range of choices that could contribute to solutions is limited (or financially inaccessible). Without a broader variety of publicly supported home services and alternative residential settings, nursing homes too soon become the only option.

Although some of the current nursing home population would be better served in alternative residential settings, persons with severe dementia, inadequate community-based support systems, and difficult-to-manage behaviors need the professionally managed care environments that these institutions are expected to provide. However, the negative images they evoke along with known inadequacies underscore the importance of continuing efforts to improve residents' quality of care and daily living conditions. Each nursing home needs to find the combination of ways that best matches its abilities to create and sustain meaningful changes. For example, increased staffing ratios and in-service education as well as utilization of advanced nurse practitioners are ways to improve quality of care. And quality of life may be improved through applying aspects of culture change philosophy such as those advanced by *The Eden Alternative* (Thomas, 1994, 1996, 1999 and http://www.edenalt.com) and *The Pioneer Network* (Lustbader, 2001 and http://www.pioneernetwork.net).

In particular, greater attention needs to be focused on the large population of residents with dementia (60–80%) whose remaining abilities and tolerances may be severely tested and confusion exacerbated by the nursing home experience (R. A. Kane et al., 1998, p. 171). As noted earlier, some nursing homes have special care units (SCUs) to accommodate selected residents. However, the pros and cons of SCUs continue to be debated. On the one hand, some residents seem to relax and function better in these environments, and persons without dementia may be equally relieved by their removal to another area. On the other hand, SCU space can accommodate only a fraction of a facility's dementia population. And concerns have been raised about (a) isolating residents with dementia from the potentially positive influences of interactions with cognitively intact residents and (b) the disruptions of personal attachments that occur when residents in decline have to transfer out of SCUs that cannot support aging in place.

Managing dementia care in congregate living settings is complicated by the inevitable juxtaposition of individual and organizational needs. Nursing home staff spend enormous amounts of time dealing with the consequences of mass housing, scheduling, and programming that, on an individual level, place all residents at a disadvantage. For example, roommate difficulties across most facilities are an almost daily occurrence that diverts staff from other work in order to "put out fires". Yet there has been too little questioning of the absurdity of forcing adults in such an individualistic society to endure this degree of intimacy (R. A. Kane et al., 1998). There are, of course, instances of close friendships between roommates and situations of peaceful coexistence or mutual avoidance. However, the degree to which persons with dementia can tolerate or be tolerated by others under these conditions is variable and often problematic.

Departmental and individual scheduling practices that govern the timing and execution of ordinary resident activities (e.g., rising, eating, socializing, going to bed) do not conform to individuals' personal rhythms and preferred daily patterns. The tyrannies of regimentation have received the most consistent public criticism and, therefore, have become a focus of innovation in many nursing homes. Often, however, frontline staff members have limited freedom to work around existing operational structures and time schedules traditionally used to allow large institutions to function efficiently and cost effectively. Thus, the nature and degree of residents' choices over matters determining their daily schedules and activities are tied to facility operations and individual staff member needs to complete work assignments. Residents with dementia are able to make choices but often need more time than an inflexible schedule and/or heavy caregiver work schedule can comfortably allow.

Finally, programming of social activities on a group scale continues to be the major means of delivering services associated with goals to increase functional abilities and address concerns about quality of life. Often the logistics of who participates depends on availability of time and resources to help residents prepare to attend and to transport them to events. Residents with dementia who require the most preparation time, give fewer or more subtle indications of the extent to which they appreciate activities, and sometimes fear to leave the unit or attend alone often are left out. For this reason, some institutions are beginning to balance community-wide activities with smaller scale unit-based and individually focused activities. This combination provides more options and is especially beneficial for persons with dementia.

In general, frontline staff members are constrained by the extent to which available human resources and administrative policies determine existing patterns of housing, scheduling, and programming in a facility. Advocates of nursing home culture change suggest that giving staff more control over their own lives through involvement in team processes, self-scheduling, and care planning "in turn enhances their capacity to ensure that residents remain decision makers in their own care" (Lustbader, 2001, p. 189). The benefit to residents with dementia will not be realized, however, unless there is a strong concurrent emphasis on better educating staff members to the environmental necessities and the simplified, undemanding conditions that foster better exercise of autonomy in this population. It has been suggested that one thing that makes SCUs "special" is "the training and skills of their staff" (R. A. Kane et al., 1998, p. 171). This is a troublesome commentary on the preparation of nursing home staff as a whole to meet the needs of the majority of residents with dementia who do not reside on SCUs.

Overall, the nursing home experience for persons with dementia varies according to how well an individual facility is prepared to meet their special needs and the nature of the needs themselves as persons progress through different stages of the disease. Others may judge what constitutes a better or poorer experience, but the only ones who truly know are the residents. Residents with dementia cannot always describe what they feel in words; but they communicate in many ways what brings joy and contentment, what brings sadness and distress, and what makes for a good or a disappointing day. In addition, their stories confirm that they have not been different from anyone else in their desires to avoid admission to a nursing home for as long as possible. Therefore, the urgency of rebalancing the long-term care system in favor of greater support for in-home services and alternative living situations cannot be stressed enough. However, nursing homes are a critical link in the chain of long-term care and when the time comes to make the decision to move into one, we all want them to be reliable sources of safe, expert care as well as nicer places in which to live.

3

Ethics in Action

OVERVIEW

This chapter discusses the meaning of ethics in action as a practical approach to understanding issues that arise in human interaction. First, it focuses on what counts as an ethical matter and suggests that moral concerns extend beyond major social conflicts, public policy struggles, and life and death issues to ordinary daily happenings that more typically affect persons who live and work in nursing homes. Second, attention turns to the application of ethics in practice. This includes perceptions about the nature and intent of ethical deliberation as well as different analytic approaches that may be used. A pluralistic appreciation of different approaches with an emphasis on practical reasoning is encouraged. Third, contextual considerations that affect the understanding of resident-focused cases are discussed as they relate to the work world of staff, organizational subcultures, and universal moral concerns. Finally, frameworks for thinking about practical resident-focused issues are offered as ways to facilitate assessment, from an ethical point of view, of the situations institutionalized persons with dementia encounter.

In the context of this discussion, ethics in action is a practical way of thinking about morality in everyday life. It assumes that all human interactions have ethical features, involving ideas about how things ought to be. These may be evident when questions or disagreements arise over the best course of action to take. But when persons are occupied in ordinary activities of everyday life, awareness of the value-driven moral aspects of individual actions and convictions may not be as high. In nursing homes, even problematic care issues may be part of what is viewed as usual and expected. Therefore, a perspective on life that asks what moral issues are at stake in every human situation may be confronted by narrower definitions of what counts as an ethical matter and also may be constrained by different views about the application of ethics in practice.

WHAT COUNTS AS AN ETHICAL MATTER?

PRACTICAL ETHICS—APPLIED AND "EVERYDAY"

The field of ethics has two main, interrelated branches. The theoretical branch (metaethics) is the domain of philosophers and professional ethicists. It encompasses the intellectual history, language, and schools of thought that provide the foundations for ethical discussions and debates. The applied branch attracts an interdisciplinary mix of people (e.g., philosophers, ethicists, practitioners, lay people, theologians, and social scientists) involved in particular fields (e.g., health care, jurisprudence, and business) for the purpose of addressing pragmatic issues that demand understanding and timely solutions. For example, historically, the place of applied ethics in health care has undergone a steady evolution. Although the first English text entitled Medical Ethics was published by Percival in 1803 (Leake, 1975), prior to the mid-20th century, public attention was not drawn to this field, the main concerns of which were focused on establishing standards of professional conduct and rules of self-regulation. In the 1960s, however, advances in modern medicine's ability to prolong life coupled with moral concerns about euthanasia and the medical experiments of Nazi Germany led to an accelerated interest within and outside of the medical profession in discussing problematic issues affecting doctor-patient relationships. Subsequently, the field of bioethics, arising in the late 1950s to the 1970s, encompassed medical ethics within a wider circle of disciplines related to "life sciences" (e.g., biology and the environment, population, and social sciences; Boyd, Higgs, & Pinching, 1997). Today, bioethics is a term that may be used interchangeably with discipline-specific terms (e.g., medical ethics, nursing ethics), or more inclusive, neutral terms (e.g., health care ethics) to denote a focus on debates, education, research, and policy initiatives associated with moral problems affecting human health and well-being. Typically, the moral problems that capture the attention of everyone are striking examples of life-and-death issues (e.g., choice in dying, euthanasia, abortion, organ transplantation), social conflict (e.g., intergenerational tensions over distribution of scarce resources), and new and emerging concerns at the forefront of scientific advances (e.g., cloning, the human genome project, experiments in genetic therapies). However, research in the field of aging has revealed a wider set of issues, grounded in the life experiences of the elderly, their families, and caregivers. A major example is R. A. Kane and Caplan's (1990) use of the anthropologically oriented notion of "everyday ethics" to encourage a broadening of concern inclusive of the ordinary moral dilemmas that touch the lives of nursing home residents on a daily basis. They argue that, although problems with roommates, personal routines, meals, and use of public and private space lack the drama of the major ethical issues of the day, they are major issues for the residents. Thus, mundane daily concerns that predominate in nursing home life need to take their place alongside of the life and death issues and policy debates that also arise in these settings.

LABELING—"WE DEAL WITH THESE ISSUES ALL THE TIME"

Every culture uses folk taxonomies (labeling schemes) in communicating about naturally occurring situations and happenings that persons encounter on a regular basis. For example, common frames of reference used in nursing homes (and worded from a caregiver point of view) are "behavior issues" (concerns about residents' difficult to manage actions); "treatment issues" (concerns about physical care and treatment); and "resource issues" (challenges involving scarcity and need). However, not all questions or decisions about the best course of action to take will be classified as ethical in nature. The most difficult cases, that are said to "rise to the top" of their categories (i.e., resist resolution), in time, may be identified as ethical dilemmas (Powers, 2000). But the ethical components of everyday interactions with residents subsumed within these ways of thinking may be taken for granted. For example, unspoken ethical considerations that often influence what people do include values related to quality of life and respect for human dignity; prioritization of competing goods and possible harms; and recognition of rights and obligations, truth and trust, fair treatment, and fair allocation of resources.

> One nurse explains: "We deal with these issues all the time. We're so used to dealing with them I'm not sure we stop often enough to really think about them."

Thus, identification of ethical issues relies, in part, on whether situations are labeled or classified as value-neutral or value-laden (Powers, 2001). That is, it is a matter of perspective that either views a course of events as ordinary and "taken-for-granted reality supported by taken-for-granted truths" or as containing an ethical aspect worthy of consideration (Kitwood, 1998, p. 24).

APPLICATION OF ETHICS IN PRACTICE

NEGATIVE ASSOCIATION—"OH DEAR! I DIDN'T KNOW THAT [THE HOME] HAD ETHICAL PROBLEMS."

The scope of ethical discussions also may be limited by perceptions about their intent. Ethical reflection does not involve presuppositions about what may be good, bad, right or wrong about a situation. But persons may be sensitized to the use of the term "ethics" in connection with reports of unethical or immoral behavior. This negative association with the idea of ethical consultation or review is reflected in a family member's comment on learning about the existence of a nursing home ethics committee.

> *"Oh dear! I didn't know that [the home] had ethical problems. I always thought they did such a good job."*

"This mistaken impression of ethics consultation as an investigation of possible wrongdoing is reinforced by newspaper accounts of the role of the ethics committee in the political arena" (J. Spike, personal communication, April, 25, 2002). Staff could have similar preconceptions about ethical consultations/reviews as well. There might be fear that examination of issues will be conducted from a critical moral perspective with conclusions handed down in the form of judgments. Persons who associate ethics with judgment and criticism will be focused on avoidance and self-protection. However, a dispassionate and respectful ethical evaluation will allow for acceptance and synthesis of different points of view. The aim is to try to understand paths of reasoning that influence people's perspectives on a matter in order to consider best ways to move ahead. Different analytic approaches may be used to sort out issues and guide recommendations (not judgments) about what to do in a given situation.

DIFFERENT ANALYTIC APPROACHES

Principlism

The practice of applying moral principles to support philosophical arguments and address real life dilemmas is the result of widespread use of the thinking outlined by Beauchamp and Childress (1983) in *Principles of Biomedical Ethics*. In their model, key principles involved in ethical analysis are: (a) autonomy (self-determination and freedom of choice); (b) beneficence (doing good and putting others' interests first); (c) nonmaleficence (doing no harm and avoiding negligence that leads to harm); (d) justice (fairness in the treatment of others); (e) fidelity (faithfulness, including honoring of covenants and promise-keeping); and (f) veracity (truth-telling, honesty, and integrity). Although principlism probably is the best known approach, it has come under significant criticism. First, many believe that a rigid preoccupation with rules and principles as a primary means of justifying moral action does not allow for adequate recognition of the complexity and diversity of human experience (Evans, 2000). That is, using a priori law-like principles as a way to insure that similar cases are treated in the same way offers less room for exercise of discretion in dealing with problematic situations than does judicious use of an individualized case-by-case approach (Toulmin, 1981). Second, the tendency to award autonomy first place in a hierarchy of articulated values (moral goods) also has raised cries for balance between rights of individuals and the competing claims of community-focused values, citizenship, duties of individuals, and the principle of distributive justice (Callahan, 1984; Danis & Churchill, 1991; Emson, 1995). Third, critics call for interpretations of principles that are based on contextual understanding of the cultural experiences and human relationships to which they apply. For example, Pellegrino and Thomasma (1988) have argued for different ways to view autonomy in illness situations where patient's decisional capacities vary and where beneficence (acting in the patient's best interests) may in some instances be the greater moral good. "At the very least, negotiation about the good to be achieved ought to take place explicitly. It should be apparent to everyone what is the 'treatment plan'" (Thomasma, 1995, p. 21).

Casuistry

Casuistry is case ethics, or ethical case analysis. In practice, it involves analyzing ethical dilemmas by comparing them to those found in previously experienced cases with satisfactory outcomes. In this way, resolution of complex cases may be guided by simple illustrations (paradigm examples) of what was helpful in cases with similar characteristics. Previous cases may be conceptualized as groupings that come together in a practical working taxonomy (classification scheme) that supports sorting out what the unique features of a particular case may be as well as what it holds in common with cases that in some ways resemble it. Jonsen and Toulmin (1988) explain:

> . . . anyone who has occasion to consider moral issues in actual detail knows that morally significant differences between cases can be as significant as their likenesses. We need to respect not only the general principles that require us to treat similar cases alike but also those crucial distinctions that justify treating dissimilar cases differently. One indispensable instrument for helping to resolve moral problems in practice, therefore, is a detailed and methodical map of morally significant likenesses and differences: what may be called a moral taxonomy. (p. 14)

Because this method places value on the uniqueness of each situation, the primary focus is that of laying out the facts of the case. Application of general ethical theories or principles plays a secondary role in explaining the basis of moral choices, that is, serving to ground the approach by illuminating values or moral goods that are inductively derived from case description. A norm in practice disciplines such as law, ethics, and health care, is that case-bound generalizations about lessons learned that may be useful in resolving future cases contribute to a growing fund of knowledge about particular topics that have been resolved successfully (Davis, 1991; Sandelowski, 1996).

Narrative Ethics

Narrative ethics, as a method of case interpretation, is closely linked to casuistry. The emphasis is on analyzing ethical dilemmas by describing a person's life story, significant experiences, and personal values as a historical sequence with a logical order that helps to explain what would be an apt final chapter. This type of storytelling approach is not a simple reconstruction of the facts of a case. Rather, it is an effort to recreate, from various participants' points of view, what living through the experience feels like in order to enable a deeper understanding of who the actors are and what has brought them to the problematic situation. It also involves imagining what future ways of moving ahead are possible and "how values and obligations can guide particular people facing complex problems to solutions that are morally justifiable" (Walker,

1993, p. 36). Hermeneutic or phenomenological methods may be used to explore the meanings that involved persons attach to a situation. By contextualizing ethical principles in this manner "one transforms a logical dilemma into one that is more readily understood as a human drama" (J. Spike, personal communication, April 25, 2002).

Descriptive Ethics

The interpretations of "sociologists, anthropologists, psychologists, historians, and others" who portray human cultures and experiences in narrative styles that attempt to capture moral behavior and concerns are linked with ethics, although ethicists would not claim descriptive ethics as a true division of their field (Fowler & Levine-Ariff, 1987, p. 27). Qualitative research traditions more readily serve in this capacity by describing situations governing human behavior and interaction in a nonvalue laden (non-normative) way that provides a context for later analysis of ethical issues. Within this genre, however, there are interpretive qualitative approaches with somewhat different aims and methods. Interpretive descriptions also establish a context to support the understanding of moral issues that arise in given situations. But work in this area of research falls more explicitly within a normative (value-laden) paradigm that does tend to produce informed (data-based) perspectives on moral issues. Interpretive sciences fit Bellah's description of "practical social science" that "overlaps with philosophy and shares many of its concerns" (Bellah, 1982, p. 38). Descriptive and interpretive accounts allow readers to make connections between reported experiences of others and their own. Discussions of issues embedded in the descriptions/interpretations suggest ways to think about them. For example, anthropological/ethnographic studies of everyday nursing home life have examined many issues from residents' points of view, e.g., privacy and personal space issues; loss of dignity and autonomy; infantilization and depersonalization; social relationship issues; victimization; reciprocity and control; problems with restraints; mealtime concerns; difficulties with routines and receiving care; and issues around death and dying (Gubrium, 1975, 1993, 1995; Kayser-Jones, 1981, 1991, 1992, 1996, 1997, 2000; Kayser-Jones, Davis, Wiener, & Higgens, 1989; O'Brien, 1989; Powers, 1988b, 1991, 1992, 1995, 1996, 1997; Savishinsky, 1991, 1995; Shield, 1988, 1995; Vesperi, 1983; Watson & Maxwell, 1977). Less often, issues from staff member points of view also have been discussed, for example, autonomy and social relationship issues; nature of and attitudes toward work; abuse of staff by residents; caregiving dilemmas and burnout; problems with bureaucracy; devaluing and dehumanization;

and turnover (Foner, 1994a, 1994b, 1995; Gubrium, 1975; Henderson, 1981, 1987, 1995; Savishinsky, 1991; Shield, 1988). Foner's work in particular has focused on the work experiences of nursing assistants. The use of cultural description to illuminate issues such as the above is a hallmark of ethnographic research. In these reports, the voices of persons whose lives are the focus of study combined with firsthand field observations of the researcher bring a richness of human experience to discussion of moral concerns.

ACCOMMODATING DIVERSITY IN MORAL DELIBERATIONS

Knowledge without understanding is useless. An appreciation of pluralism opens the door to the richness and strengths of different approaches. There are concerns, however, that such openness also involves risk of ethical deliberation becoming too relativistic, that is, belief that, since there are many perspectives on what is true, right, or good, there are no universal criteria—only different perspectives—on such matters (Boyd et al., 1997, p. 216). This, itself, is an extreme view (and, as these authors point out, is, ironically, only one perspective)! Some might argue that rigid adherence to principlism represents another extreme, that is, that it is a method designed to simplify ethical decision-making by reducing/discarding notions of complexity (e.g., individual complexity, different perspectives, situational context) and condensing morality down to central, easily grasped elements (Evans, 2000, p. 32). "Principlism neglects the moral life and moral character of the various agents involved; these are treated as so much 'noise' or error variance to be factored out of the ethical equation" (Hofland, 2001, p. 26).

A moderate view calls for balance, respect, and reflexivity lest human lives become entangled in academic debates. In active practice, theoretical concepts and traditional methods of principle-based ethics and casuistry are useful tools, but they are not enough. Practical ethics also needs the detailed substance of human experience that descriptive and narrative approaches use to help bring people's stories to life and place individual cases in meaningful contexts.

Ethics in action moves back and forth between two poles—one that summarizes moral goods (principles and values) and the other that attempts to understand human situations—everyday concerns as well as life and death issues—in all their complexities (contextualization). It also emphasizes practical reasoning—Aristotelian "deliberation which gives equal weight to what one ought to do morally and what one can do in practice, and which leads to a decision and effective action" (Boyd et al., 1997, p. 192).

CONTEXTUAL CONSIDERATIONS

In nursing home settings, issues of everyday life tend to predominate. Therefore, ability to understand resident-focused concerns depends upon developing perspectives about common social and cultural contexts that shape their daily experiences. Those discussed below include the work world of staff and the organizational subcultures within which that work is accomplished. Moral concerns that emanate from these aspects of nursing home culture have implications for preserving and respecting the personhood of both residents and staff.

THE WORK WORLD OF STAFF—"YOU KNOW, WE'RE HUMAN"

Moral dilemmas do not occur in a vacuum. Therefore, concerns about ethical treatment of nursing home residents must take into account the social organization in which those concerns arise. For example, when individual residents' cases are presented, details about how the management of their care fits within the workloads of nursing home staff cannot be glossed over or omitted. This involves a need to know persons who care for the resident and to understand the nature of their work. There are many categories of personnel whose interactions with residents ought to be considered. However, attention in the literature and popular press often is focused on certified nursing assistants (CNAs) who deliver most of the personal physical care that nursing home residents receive. Therefore, their work world will be the focus here.

On the day shift, each CNA may have seven, eight, or more individuals for whom he/she primarily is responsible. There always will be a certain amount of rushing that has to take place in the morning (around residents that CNAs know really cannot be rushed). Persons need to be helped out of bed, toileted, bathed, groomed, and dressed in time for breakfast, appointments, and the many other activities of the day. Day shift CNAs serve and assist residents with two meals, make beds, change soiled clothing and bed linens, help each other when more than one person is needed, and repeat many of the same forms of assistance for multiple individuals throughout the shift.

Nurse: When you think about it, they have seven-and-a-half hours of work. They have to take at least two-and-a-half hours a day to feed [residents].

And they have to toilet everybody every two to four hours, give morning care, do all the beds, clean all the rooms. . . . There isn't enough time . . .

Evening shift staff are fewer in number and may work in teams to serve and assist with the evening meal, give baths to some residents, and prepare persons for bedtime. Night shift is the most sparsely staffed in nursing homes, on the premise that there is no need to be readying residents for meals and activities during these hours when most of them are expected to be sleeping. However, residents with dementia, in particular, may be restless and wakeful at night. And many residents are incontinent or need to be taken to the bathroom. Thus, this typical staffing pattern stretches resources if there are a number of residents who are ill, wakeful, or up and about at the same time. Overall, on every shift, the work is tiring, emotionally stressful, and physically demanding with bending, lifting, and holding up persons who are unable to move and support themselves or to control their bodily functions and behavior.

Staff, and CNAs in particular, may be abused by residents who scream at and insult them as well as scratch, spit, bite, slap, kick, or punch. Generally, staff will say that they understand that they cannot take such behavior on the part of residents with dementia personally, but this is not an easy or comfortable proposition.

Nurse: They [residents] just say things [swearing and insults] and you can't let it bother you; but it's very difficult for some people to take. I've been called all kinds of things. And no matter how you tell yourself—'They don't mean me. It's just part of their disease'—it's difficult, [and] it can be so devastating to [some people]. You can tell [who should not be assigned to certain residents] by the way they interact. Some people just can't [protect themselves emotionally from continuous verbal abuse] and talk with a smile in their voice all the time.

Sometimes staff members, knowledgeable of residents' ways, wait for a change of mood.

CNA: "You never know when [Mrs. C's] going to be angry or not angry. [When she's angry] she will bite you, she'll hit you, and she'll kick you. She doesn't want anybody to touch her. I leave her alone [and] she gets over it pretty quick . . . I've had her on my assignment for about six years."

At other times persons accept abuse as part of the job and persevere.

Family member: "[The CNA] was changing her in the bathroom and . . . Oh! She hit her so hard. I wanted to die. But [the CNA] just said, 'I'm used to it,' and continued on and got her changed. I couldn't do it."

Individuals respond differently to the physical and emotional demands of their work. One CNA comments on the diversity of the workforce and expresses the need for cohesion and supportive relationships among staff in order for them to be effective. This implies that staff also need times alone together to strengthen personal bonds and assess their feelings about the working situations that they share.

"We all are not the same. We're not going to act the same and have the same values . . . [And with] a lot to do, and you've got so little time . . . Anybody can have a bad day. [But] if we have differences, we can pull each other aside and talk about how we feel. Because if you're upset, your mind won't be on your work; and then the residents are not going to get the kind of care they need. [And for a job well done] . . . it doesn't hurt to have a compliment once in awhile."

Another nursing assistant finds that taking "time out" when tension builds is an important and helpful thing to do.

"You know, we're human. I mean, the residents get frustrated sometimes. Well, the aides do too. But you have to know when to say, 'I have to step off for a second and take a break off the floor.' And that helps . . . to go off the floor for a few moments and come back. Then you're ready to start over. By the time you come back, maybe the situation has changed completely."

Nursing home staff members are unique individuals themselves. They are human and their work world is challenging. In addition, they are repeatedly confronted by nationally publicized cases of nursing home abuse of residents by staff. The factual and harrowing nature of these reports shakes public confidence in nursing homes and shapes opinions about workers, nursing assistants in particular. For competent, caring nursing home staff, it is an added but necessary burden—necessary from the point of view of needed vigilance and moral accountability for reporting abuse and mistreatment by those individuals who should not be entrusted with the care of other people.

ORGANIZATIONAL SUBCULTURES

A single institution may support noticeably different subcultures across its residential living units that influence ways in which CNAs approach their work. For example, the following comments contrast work patterns on a particular special care unit for persons with dementia and other units in the same facility. On the special care unit, strategies for dividing time between residents typically are devised and modified, based on knowledge of individual needs and tolerances.

> *"[Mr. A] can be happy or headstrong. Sometimes he's the father figure and wants it [care] done right then. Then some days he's really unpleasant; and some days he sleeps quite a bit. I have to let him have his way. When I approach and say 'Good morning,' if he says 'Good morning' back, I know everything's kinda calm. But if not, he doesn't want to be bothered with early. I'll just tell him I'm coming back later, and then he'll calm down. Then I go back to him [and] I try as many times as possible, however long I'm here that day. Now [Mr. B] is totally different. He likes it when you're persistent with him. You just keep nudging him on and on and on, and eventually he'll cooperate with you. So [the approach to him is] totally different. Some days, the first three residents I usually do in the morning may be asleep, so I let them sleep. Then some days [Mr. A's]ready to get done at 7:30. I never know what to expect when I come in; so I have to be prepared to deal with whatever's going on. Their moods change quite a bit and you have to learn to adjust."*

In the above setting, the philosophy of care fosters a more flexible approach in recognition of residents' needs and in acknowledgement of practical experience that shows these individuals to be least "programmable." In fact, unwillingness to accept imposed daily routines to the point of being disruptive may be an element in decisions to transfer an individual from a regular floor to a special care unit.

> *A wife explains: It was a good move [to the special care unit] because I think they [the residents] were more restricted on the [other] floor. They had a certain time for putting them to bed and getting them up for breakfast. And they were wonderful people, but he's a stubborn man. He even kicked and punched because when he didn't want to do something, he wasn't going to do it. [On the special care unit] they [residents] make their own schedule, and the staff kinda caters to their schedule. And I noticed he's much, much calmer here than on the [other] floor.*

Management styles may be influenced by the nature of the resident population. For example, in this scenario, residents on the special care unit may evidence a variety of behaviors that are difficult to deal with on a general resident unit. But still, they are more homogeneous than the resident mix on other units. Other units have a more diverse mix of residents. There will be residents with mild to moderate dementia and some remaining functional abilities that need time and assistance in getting through the day. And there will be residents who are totally dependent and require complete physical care, often involving time-consuming treatments. Some of the latter will be very ill or dying. Their needs for physical care and emotional support will be complex. One way to see that care of this broad range of resident needs is managed safely and efficiently is to impose a structured routine that everyone on staff can follow. There also will be residents who appreciate and find security in any known routine. The difficulty lies with those who, needing more flexibility, do not benefit from it.

> *Special care unit nurse: "On the other units, I think [staff] are used to being able to do things according to their schedule . . . and when [residents] don't fit in that schedule, it's very difficult for them . . . because they don't have the time for it. They're task-oriented. They have all these things that have to be accomplished and such little time . . . It's a mind set."*

The special care unit in this nursing home transfers most residents who become totally dependent and require complete care to other floors. If it did not, it would develop more of a diverse resident mix as well, and, arguably, would be less able to function in the flexible manner that it does.

> *Special care unit nurse: "It's very difficult for the staff to take people that have regressed so that they're total care . . . very difficult care [that involves] a lot of medical interventions. And . . . I mean, these people are our family; we're really connected to them . . . But we can't have it both ways. We can't have such a heavy caseload that the nursing assistants can't deal with the dementia problems and the behavior problems."*

These brief examples suggest that external organizational factors as well as individual ability and style influence the manner in which nursing assistants carry out their work. All have implications for residents and their care. Therefore, any resident-centered ethical dilemma will need to be approached with an understanding of the work management strategies and philosophies that underlie delivery of care and services in a particular nursing home as well as on various units in a facility (given that there are bound to be differences).

UNIVERSAL MORAL CONCERNS

The external and internal diversity of nursing homes does not preclude the identification of some fundamental moral concerns that apply to all. First, there is the *concern for avoiding harm and providing exemplary care to residents.* The current nursing home population mainly consists of frail, ill persons in need of sophisticated clinical care and considerable physical assistance. There is no doubt that some resident care issues (including rushing residents, shortcuts and cutting corners, unsafe practices, neglect and abuse) may be traced to circumstances where staff are not sufficiently trained and/or are pressed for time to meet the needs of the number of residents assigned to them. This concern has been affirmed by a panel of experts whose recommendations for minimum staffing standards are based on government data showing that average levels of nursing staff (nurses and nursing assistants) providing direct care in nursing homes are inadequate (Harrington et al., 2000). Benefits to residents (and nursing home inspection outcomes) accrue from a combination of reducing workloads of direct care providers, utilizing the expertise of advanced practice nurses, and increasing the emphasis on staff member education and effective nursing management strategies to raise quality of care.

Second, there is the concern for *recognizing and dealing with competition between organizational and individual interests.* Some resident care issues have organizational causes. Organizational factors that have an impact on resident care include staffing, scheduling, and management of various departments; internal interpersonal or departmental conflicts; availability and distribution of goods and services; policies/rules/regulations; and business office practices. However, it is difficult to talk about solutions that might involve changing problem-producing aspects of an institution's structure or organizational culture as long as the issues themselves continue to be seen as individual resident-centered ethical dilemmas. There needs to be a willingness to identify and address institutional policies, practices, and other internal matters that affect quality of care and quality of life. Shifting from a microlevel focus on individual resident cases to a macrolevel focus on nursing home organization and culture accomplishes this end.

Third, there is the *concern for preserving and respecting personhood.* Personhood includes a subjective sense of one's individuality (*personal identity*) and one's social connections with other people (*social identity*), forged and refined in the context of human interaction. For example, Kitwood's (1998) categorization of interactions that affect the personhood of individuals with dementia is summarized below.

Actions That Maintain Personhood

Recognition (calling persons by name, eye contact); *Negotiation* (asking about their preferences, wishes, and needs); *Collaboration* (doing things *with,* not *to* persons); *Play, Timalation [sic/neologism], and Celebration* (encouraging spontaneity, providing reassuring contact, and connecting spiritually); *Relaxation, Validation, and Holding* (projecting calm acceptance, acknowledging emotions and feelings, promoting trust); *Facilitation, Creation, and Giving* (enabling persons to successfully initiate actions/interactions, praising their helpfulness, and showing sincere appreciation for their expressions of affection or concern for self and others).

Actions That Undermine Personhood

Treachery (using deception and manipulation to force compliance); *Disempowerment* (not allowing or helping persons to use the abilities they do have); *Infantilization* (patronizing or treating persons as children); *Intimidation* (using threats or physical force); *Labeling and Stigmatization* (belittling, devaluing); *Outpacing* (communicating too rapidly for persons to understand and rushing them); *Invalidation* (failing to acknowledge persons' feelings and understandings about reality as they perceive it); *Banishment, Objectification, and Ignoring* (excluding persons, treating them as if they had no thoughts or feelings, and acting in their presence as if they were not there); *Imposition, Withholding, and Accusation* (denying choice, refusing to give attention/neglecting, blaming persons for what results from their lack of ability or misunderstandings); *Disruption, Mockery, and Disparagement* (interrupting/intruding, teasing/making fun of or humiliating persons).

The assumption is that persons with dementia, regardless of the severity of their cognitive impairment, have valid personal identities, meaning-driven behavior, and feelings that can be affected by the behavior of other people around them (Kitwood, 1998; Post, 2000b; Sabat, 1998). But ordinary daily patterns of interaction are part of "the taken for granted world [that] most of the time . . . exists below the threshold of awareness;" and, therefore, the moral nature of individuals' everyday exchanges often is not "brought forward for detailed and unprejudiced examination" (Kitwood, 1998, p. 30). It is important to add that the above actions described as constituting support or lack of support of personhood apply in every type of social situation. Consequently, a natural conclusion is that, in nursing homes, concern for how individuals are treated cannot be limited to residents. Applying Kitwood's observations about how persons are affected by the way they are treated on a broader scale involves also recognizing the personhood of nursing home staff as a serious moral obligation. Simply put, if nursing home residents are to be treated with respect, kindness, and understanding, then nursing home staff must be treated that way as well. Nursing home cultures that are committed to respecting moral personhood in human relationships at all organizational levels are better positioned to deliver high quality care and to think about ways to create more desirable social and daily living environments.

FRAMEWORKS FOR ASSESSING RESIDENT-FOCUSED ISSUES

To briefly summarize before moving on—*Chapter 1: Living with Dementia* describes people's pre-nursing home experiences, based on the retrospective accounts of family members. Consideration of some characteristic concerns about getting help for cognitively impaired persons and dealing with problems in daily living provides a foundation for understanding the nature of the disease and its effects on people in the time leading up to nursing home admission. The shift in personal orientation from a community-based context to the organizational context described in *Chapter 2: The Nursing Home Experience* represents a major life change for residents and their families. Despite the important role they play in the long-term care system, nursing homes are not a preferred residential option for most people. Some previously enjoyed autonomy is relinquished. Persons with dementia become "residents." Family caregivers become their "advocates." And the organizational culture of a particular nursing home setting becomes the orienting framework for dealing with concerns about the quality of personal care, social relationships, and daily living environments. *Chapter 3: Ethics in Action* combines views on what counts as an ethical matter and particular contexts that shape how moral concerns are understood with information about recognized styles of ethical analysis. Ethics in Action is described as subscribing to a pluralistic approach that emphasizes practical reasoning. Discussion of contextual considerations that shape resident experiences precedes discussion of frameworks for resident-focused case analysis.

Any framework that is helpful in organizing needed elements of a case to promote discussion and action will serve. Two are described. The one that is used to present illustrative cases in this book is a research-based taxonomy of ways to think about ethical issues that affect nursing home residents with dementia (Powers, 2001). Its compatibility with what Jonsen et al. (1998) identify as important in clinical case analysis is discussed.

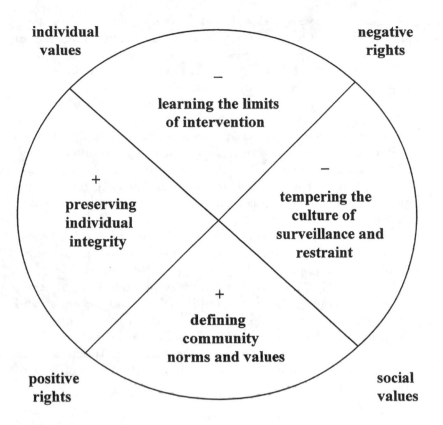

FIGURE 3.1   Taxonomy of everyday ethical issues.

Originally published by Bethel Ann Powers in *Nursing Research, 50*, 332–339, 2001, Ethnographic analysis of everyday ethics in the care of nursing home residents with dementia: A taxonomy. Used with the permission of Lippincott, Williams, & Wilkins.

A TAXONOMY OF EVERYDAY ETHICAL ISSUES

The taxonomy of everyday ethical issues (Fig. 3.1) includes four domains that are oriented toward individual and social values (Powers, 2001). These intersecting planes summarize ethical concerns that commonly arise in institutional cultures. Positive and negative valences associated with each domain represent distinctions between positive moral rights (the rights to have something done for or given to an individual) and negative moral rights (the rights not to have something done to or taken from an individual). Dimensions of the taxonomy are described below. Hypothetical examples are based on real experiences that have been altered and blended to respect confidentiality and limit them to description of the issues of interest rather than actual persons from whom they were derived. Suggestions on ways to orient discussion in cases readers might encounter that contain similar or different issues than those in the examples are based on the following ideas:

- *Examining institutional policies* may help clarify specific situations or lead to suggestions for new or clearer policies. In addition to formal written policies, there may be unwritten practices/ways of doing things that are treated as policies or rules. Focusing on standard operating procedures can explain an issue or lead to changes that resolve it.
- *Searching for meaning in residents' actions* involves considering factors that may influence their responses and help to explain how a situation might appear to them.
- *Evaluating the role dementia plays* involves estimating what cognitive impairment contributes to residents' actions and responses and how it may affect approaches to resolution of issues and concerns.
- *Consulting related sources* on identified issues revealed by actual cases can enrich discussion and support recommendations. These could be articles, reports, films, or other works that shed light on experiences in dementia care.

DIMENSIONS OF THE TAXONOMY

Individual and Social Values

Individual Values—Two domains focus on individual values, calling attention to concerns about respect for residents' personal rights and individuality. *Learning the limits of intervention* involves people's negative moral rights, such as the right not to be forced to do things. Forcing includes using threats, fear, and intimidation to obtain compliance; manipulating or tricking/deceiving people into following one's wishes; or depriving them of something in exchange for their cooperation.

> *Example #1: At times, Mrs. A is very aggressive when staff attempt to give care (bathing, dressing, toileting). She kicks, scratches, and bites. In extreme situations, staff have an order for an injection (psychotropic medication) to calm her, but they sometimes are fearful to administer it and also prefer to try lesser measures (going away and returning later, spending quiet*

time together, diversionary activities, alternate care approaches). Staff questions are: When a person lacks capacity, has he/she lost the right to refuse care? At what point do we intervene? At what point do we use psychotropic drugs? Do we accept the side effects of medication (i.e., lethargy) to gain the benefit (i.e., decreased agitation and combativeness)? Sometimes we need to do for residents what they cannot do for themselves. How will we communicate with family and among ourselves to establish minimum standards of care? At what point do we say that the resident has to have care? Is "forcing" always wrong?

The limits of caregivers' duties to intervene in cases where residents with dementia actively refuse and/or resist care and treatment is a frequently occurring issue. There are many worries attached to staff conversations about this topic. For example: When does respecting residents' rights to refuse care/treatment constitute neglect? How may others (e.g., family members, supervisors and other staff members, visitors, state inspectors) be expected to distinguish between legitimate concessions to residents' rights to refuse versus dereliction of duty? How do caregivers resolve feelings of frustration and guilt when resident wishes do not complement their own personal values and professional care standards? Under what circumstances, if any, is it ever justifiable to force a resident to do or submit to something against his/her will? Do all forms of force, including intimidation, manipulation, and trickery constitute abuses regardless of the circumstance? Does the end justify the means?

Discussion about particular cases might involve:

- Examining institutional policies: *Does the nursing home have written policies specifically related to residents' rights and the use of force?*
- Searching for meaning in residents' actions: *What triggers the frustration?* For example, sometimes care of a very personal nature embarrasses adults. A noisy environment, being rushed, or being left alone with a task to complete also can make people anxious. *What factors could be involved?* Fatigue, pain, discomfort, or sensory (hearing, visual) impairments can cause reactions. There may be anger over inability to verbally express wishes, needs, and feelings; to understand what others say; or to remember how to do things. There may be medical reasons such as infection, medication toxicity, a new illness or exacerbation of a chronic condition, or psychiatric issues such as depression, delusions, or hallucinations.
- Evaluating the role dementia plays: *What signs of cognitive disorder are present?* Aphasia (language impairment) affects verbal expression

and/or comprehension. Apraxia (impaired ability to do motor tasks) causes performance difficulties. Injury to some parts of the brain leads to loss of emotional control. *What abilities remain?* Persons with dementia can express wishes/needs/feelings in many ways, if not in words. Some persons respond well to simple directions, structure, routines, or reminders. *Has there been a significant change in the person's behavior?* Increase in frequency or severity of aggressive, agitated behavior or, conversely, evidence of decline should result in reassessment of progressive loss of cognition as well as for new or emerging medical, social, or environmental problems.

- Consulting related sources: *Are there specific care activities most associated with a resident's distress/resistance?* There are many practice-focused books and articles in professional journals that provide helpful tips about alternate approaches to care (e.g., bathing, dressing, management of incontinence, assistance with eating). See, for example, Kayser-Jones & Schell (1997b); Jirovec & Wells (1990); Mahoney, Volicer, & Hurley (2000); Rader (1994 & 1995); and Vogelpohl et al. (1996). The applicability of these kinds of ideas to the case at hand might enrich the discussion.

Learning the limits of intervention also may involve individuals' negative moral rights not to receive treatment against their expressed wishes.

Example #2: Mr. B's advance directives specifically request that antibiotics (among other measures) not be used to prolong his life. Since his dementia is advanced to the point where meaningful conversation is not possible, his son (designated health care proxy) requested that antibiotics being given for a respiratory infection be discontinued, stating that Mr. B had been waiting to die for some time, and treatment was not warranted. (The infection resolved without antibiotic treatment.) In contrast, Mrs. C's advance directives also request that antibiotics and other measures not be used to prolong life. As her dementia progresses, she has become increasingly anxious and frequently speaks about wanting to die, having nothing left to live for, and not wanting to continue living "like this." However, in response to her complaints of discomfort, antibiotics were used to treat a respiratory infection, from which she recovered. Questions to consider include: What influences different approaches to cases with the same written treatment preferences? Is there a difference between Mr. B's "waiting to die" and Mrs. C's "desire to die"? Is Mrs. C's expression of a desire to die actually an expression of a need for more caring attention? Is Mr. B's son as informed as he could be about his father's medical condition? How much weight is given to advance directives vs. family member opinion? Is withholding an antibiotic, which can relieve uncomfortable symptoms, equivalent to prolonging life? Is giving an antibiotic that previously was indicated as not desired disrespecting a resident's autonomy and personhood?

Caregivers' duties to intervene are constrained by stated preferences in residents' advance directives to limit life-sustaining treatments. The ethical issues these may raise often involve others' relative comfort with withholding treatment; disagreements over whether the time has come to follow the directives; unwillingness to enforce them; and uncertainty about what they really mean. For example, wishes for an absence of heroics should not result in neglect or abandonment. Kayser-Jones et al. (1989) present an excellent example of failed advocacy for a resident whose suffering and death was attributed to a neglectful family and to professional caregivers who "confused heroics with reasonable therapeutic care" (p. 269). Uncertainty also may be present in the form of questions about how informed the person's understanding was at the time, whether he/she would feel the same way now (if elicitation of wishes is difficult or impossible), what might be seen as indicators of residents' present wishes, how best to honor them, and who should decide. Discussion about particular cases might involve:

- Examining institutional policies: *What types of documentation are kept on file regarding residents' advance directives, health care proxy, power of attorney, decisions to forego life-sustaining treatment, and circumstances under which there is an agreement not to use cardiopulmonary resuscitation?* Advance directives and do-not-resuscitate (DNR) orders were described in Chapter 1 as important documents that enable individuals to indicate what treatment options they do and do not wish to have administered when it has been determined that they are in a terminal condition. In a recent issue of *The Gerontologist* (Buckwalter, Guest Editor, 2002) devoted to articles on end-of-life research with a focus on older populations, Mezey, Dubler, Mitty, and Brody (2002) report the following review of the literature findings. Documented success of skilled nursing home facilities (SNFs) in achieving high percentages of advance directives and DNR orders in place for residents (Mezey, Teresi, Ramsey, Mitty, & Bobrowitz, 2000; Tolle, Rosenfeld, Tilden, & Park, 1999) has been shown to translate into improved quality of end-of-life care and decreases in unnecessary transfers of dying persons to hospitals (Cohen-Mansfield et al., 1991). However, there also is evidence of hospital transfers occurring when families are unable to abide by advance directives that stipulate: "do not hospitalize" . . . "comfort care" . . . "palliative care only" (Travis, Loving, McClanahan, & Bernard, 2001). And, many cognitively impaired SNF residents have neither advance directive nor family/health care proxy to make decisions on their behalf (Coleman & Petruzzelli, 2001). What these findings suggest is that there is a need to educate the public about the importance of completing advance directives, especially in early stages of dementia before there is marked decline in persons' decision-making capacities. In this way, individuals entrust that when they are no longer able to make treatment decisions, their previous requests will be used as part of their treatment plans (Rempusheski & Hurley, 2000). However, even though documentation of persons' prior convictions about their health care is very helpful, it does not eliminate doubts about what their understanding of their circumstances would be at the point of decision. Doubts occur when family members/proxies making decisions on another's behalf have not had the kind of relationship that allows them to speak truly for the other and have not made a significant investment of time in discussing the issues in depth with that individual. Drought and Koenig (2002) also identify problems with focusing on an idealized conception of "choice" when the choice does not exist (choice not to die of a terminal illness) and when "the balance of power [in shared decision making] is weighted toward the clinician . . . who determines the range and possibility of patient choice by the treatment options that are offered . . . [and who is in turn] constrained by the systems within which he or she practices" (pp. 115–116).

• Searching for meaning in residents' actions: *How does the person in declining physical health and with directives to forego life-sustaining treatment respond to others' concentration on providing specific comfort measures (palliative care) and more personal attention?* Over time, desired responses may include temporary change in the direction of the decline, increased relaxation, and reduced signs of distress. *Does the person have capacity or competency to make decisions about treatments?* Decisional capacity refers to a clinical determination made by a physician about a person's ability to make decisions based on ability to communicate preferences, to understand what is being communicated, and to make a choice. Competency refers to the presumed ability and automatic right of United States citizens to make decisions, on reaching the age of adulthood. Incompetency refers to a legal determination made by a judge that a person does not have the ability to make responsible decisions.

• Evaluating the role dementia plays: *How should situations involving persons with variable/partially intact capacity be managed?* Persons with dementia may be able to make some decisions but unable to make others and, for many reasons, their abilities to make decisions may vary over the hours of a day or from day to day. Thus, additional factors in judging capacity to make a decision would include the seriousness/risks and benefits and complexity of the particular decision and the consistency of the person's expression of his/her desires with regard to that specific concern over a period of time. *What kind of support do health care proxies of persons with dementia need?* A designated proxy may be legally empowered to supply "substituted judgments" for a person who lacks capacity. But ability to function well in this role depends upon receiving clear, continuous, accurate, and complete information about the person's condition; attention to expressed concerns; answers to questions; and understanding, empathetic responses to the feelings and emotions that are a part of the family/close friend/proxy experience.

• Consulting related sources: *Are there palliative care approaches that distress or cause concerns for families and/or staff?* Recognizing when it is futile to pursue life-sustaining treatments (that many advance directives preclude) may be accompanied by emotional distress. For example, decisions not to use artificial feeding (e.g., nasogastric or gastrostomy tube) in the case of a person with severe dementia who can no longer take nourishment by mouth are difficult. Since there cannot be an absolute rule that will serve in every case, the process of weighing stated preferences to forego treatment against medical considerations and family wishes often tests personal values and feelings. But reaching a decision to honor the advance directive may not in itself eliminate caregivers' stress. Withdrawing nutritional support brings sadness as individuals struggle to accept that the person's life is ending. People ask if starvation and dehydration cause discomfort. Literature suggests that it is unlikely, going on to explain the physiologic changes that occur as death approaches (e.g., Fordyce, 2000; McCann, Hall, & Groth-Juncker, 1994; Zerwekh, 1997). Tailoring pain relief in care of persons with dementia also involves removal of barriers to professional knowledge about newest developments and guiding practice principles (Miller, Nelson, & Mezey, 2000). Kayser-Jones (2002) has further identified commonly encountered end-of-life symptoms and problems that nursing homes may need to be better prepared to assess and manage (e.g., depression, loneliness, fear, constipation, isolation, anxiety, edema, anorexia, insomnia, and fatigue). Also families, in turn, need information as well as caring support (Kayser-Jones, 2002; Mezey, Miller, & Linton-Nelson, 1999). There is a wealth of readily available material about palliative care to consult that is targeted to common end-of-life issues and oriented toward both professional care providers and family caregivers. And, in recent years, there has been some very useful development of principles and guidelines for care of people at end of life (Cassel & Foley, 1999; Lynn, 1997; Mezey et al., 2001).

Preserving the integrity of the individual involves people's positive moral rights, such as the right to respect for human dignity; appreciation of personal uniqueness and individuality; consideration of special needs for care, support, comfort and security; and freedom to do as one wishes. The latter includes making basic choices (e.g., what to eat, what to wear, etc.); managing one's time/ deciding how to order one's day; pursuing activity that satisfies one's desires and interests; and refusing invitations, if so inclined.

Example: Mr. D's morning care is extensive, since he can do nothing to assist himself and needs to be moved between bed and chair by two nursing assistants with the aid of a mechanical lift. He would prefer to eat breakfast, at the same time as other residents do, in the dining room. But his regularly assigned caregiver would not be able to see that the other five residents for whom she is responsible get to the dining room if she concentrated on Mr. D first. Presently, after breakfast in bed, he is in a wheelchair for much of the day, taking his other meals in the dining room and attending many activities. He repeatedly expresses frustration, however, over an unsatisfactory beginning to his day. He would like a different schedule, but he does not want to wake up earlier (presuming night shift workers begin his care) and he does not want a different caregiver. The care team has discussed alternatives, but each involves unpopular changes in other residents' schedules and/or caregivers. They continue to seek a compromise with Mr. D, although his dementia makes it difficult for him to understand the issues. Questions are: Do staff have the right not to honor Mr. D's request? How can they best resolve the situation to his satisfaction? How should his needs and wishes be considered in relation to those of other residents?

Discussion about particular cases might involve:

• Examining institutional policies: *What are the daily job expectations/operating procedures of staff (food service workers, nursing assistants, housekeeping) whose schedules and routines shape what a typical day is like for residents?* How staff members believe they have to organize themselves to get their work done is an important part of conversations about residents' desires for a different personal routine.

• Searching for meaning in residents' actions: *What choices is the resident able to make?* Are residents' demands communicating distress over loss of dignity and control over their lives? Giving more choices may produce fewer struggles. *Are the reasons for resident requests fully explored?* For example, what does being in the dining room for breakfast mean for Mr. D (e.g., feeling more refreshed and comfortable, enjoying the atmosphere, being with friends, etc.)? *Are alternative choices possible for residents when other requests are difficult to fulfill?* For example, could Mr. D eat breakfast in the dining room at a later time? Alternatively, what might he choose as a personal ritual to make having breakfast in his room more enjoyable (e.g., measures to promote relaxation, another person as a meal companion, his favorite music/TV show, or pet visit)?

• Evaluating the role dementia plays: *How can the resident's right to self-determination be supported?* Simple choices can be presented in a relaxed manner to residents with dementia, who often have difficulty when rushed and forced to think about more than one thing at a time. If their wishes cannot be honored, reasoning logically with them is unlikely to be effective, but offering alternatives may restore a sense of control.

• Consulting related sources: *Are there creative ways to introduce variety into the environment?* Descriptions of nursing home culture change offer many innovative ideas about ways in which nursing home environments can be transformed. This involves introducing elements of the natural environment into institutional settings in ways that produce variety, stimulate interests, support individuality, promote community, and enable residents to form more meaningful relationships with other people.

Social values—Two domains focus on social values, calling attention to concerns about duties to provide service appropriate to residents' individual and collective needs in a community context. *Tempering the culture of surveillance and restraint* involves people's negative rights not to be restrained, confined, or intruded upon.

Example: Mrs. E is a widow who recently lost her husband to Alzheimer's disease. For years, she was his devoted caregiver. Now she has begun to cultivate many friendships with other residents. But she has become especially preoccupied with Mr. Y, a widower with a diagnosis of dementia. Mr. Y leans on her for assistance, and they are almost always together.

Some residents have complained to staff about their behavior (e.g., non-sexual touching, kissing, and embracing; visits in her private room). Staff also have been asked to intervene on other residents' behalf. Specifically, some residents do not like the couple warning others away from a select table in a windowed corner of the dining room that they have chosen to claim as their own. And, Mr. Y's roommate does not like Mrs. E coming in and out of the room to help him shave and dress and to tidy up his belongings. Staff choose to express their concerns in terms of safety and care. For example, Mrs. E's preoccupation with Mr. Y causes her to disregard her own needs to use a walker for balance when ambulating and to receive assistance in maintaining a toileting routine to manage her incontinence. Mr. Y's family is not disturbed by the relationship, but Mrs. E's family members are pained by it and believe the couple should be separated. Mrs. E declares that she is an adult who can choose her own friends, and her family has no right to tell her what to do. Questions are: What should staff do about issues of surveillance and privacy? What should they do about their own feelings (i.e., values about intimate relationships between unmarried adults)? What should they do about other residents' complaints? Which values (communal or individual) should receive greater weight? What understandings should there be about use of public and private space? To what extent should family member concerns influence Mrs. E's private life? What should staff do when Mrs. E chooses to put Mr. Y's interests before her own safety and care needs?

The above example cannot reflect the whole variety of cases concerning social value-driven practices related to surveillance and/or restraint. With this understanding, discussion about particular cases containing similar or different issues might involve:

- Examining institutional policies: *What do written policies about residents' rights and residents' responsibilities say?* Residents have the right to be treated with consideration and respect for their dignity, individuality, and privacy; to have freedom of movement (freedom from restraints unless medically indicated); and to be free to associate and communicate privately with persons of their choice. As members of the nursing home community, they have a responsibility to respect the dignity and right to privacy of other residents. And they have a responsibility to cooperate with staff in following their own health care plan. *Is there a written policy concerning sexual expression and residents' needs for physical intimacy?* Such a policy would address protection of residents' rights to enjoy human companionship and intimacy (with attention to rights of residents with dementia) and would describe staff members' responsibilities to both residents and families. *Is there a specific policy concerning use of restraints?* Such a policy would explain the rationale for maintaining a restraint-free environment, the conditions under which restraints might be appropriate, and the processes used to evaluate their necessity on an ongoing basis.

• Searching for meaning in residents' actions: *What makes life worthwhile for a particular individual?* The human need for meaningful relationships is universal. What individuals desire in a relationship varies. Some persons seek opportunities to experience a sense of being valued or needed. For others, receiving attention and care from someone fills an important need. The wish to be together accompanied by expressions of warmth and affection are natural outcomes of mutually satisfying relationships. Opposite and same-sex friendships between nursing home residents occur regularly. In some cases, residents with dementia misidentify another person as a spouse. Most of the time, signs of affection and intimacy do not lead to sexual activity. However, families and staff may find any type of intimate relationship between unmarried residents distressing, especially when community-dwelling spouses are still a part of residents' lives. These are ethical matters that need to be discussed in ways that take everyone's concerns into account. But resolutions should not automatically preclude the rights of unmarried adults to satisfy their emotional and sexual needs through intimate relationships, nor disqualify residents with dementia from consideration in such matters. Homes also must meet needs for maintaining sexual relations between married couples by providing places for private visitation, learn how to accept and deal with some individuals' sexual needs for self-stimulation, and teach staff how to manage residents' inappropriate sexual behavior in ways that preserve dignity. Nursing homes cannot ignore or deny people's pursuit of self-fulfillment. In American society, adults are free to move about (a taken-for-granted right), choosing personal lifestyles and activities that make life worthwhile for them. This includes the right to decide, with other consenting adults, what the nature of relationships will be. *How do residents' communicate feelings about what is satisfying or meaningful to them?* Many residents, including those with dementia, can communicate these feelings in words. Other communications include sounds, facial expressions, gestures, and actions suggesting pleasure/displeasure about such things as being with/being removed from the company of another person, being monitored and directed by staff, being confined to a certain area, or being prevented from leaving the bed/getting up out of a chair. *In the exercise of individual rights, what considerations can others reasonably demand?* People often mistake an assault on their personal values and feelings as an intrusion on their rights. However, they cannot demand that others conform to their values or beliefs. Using the above example, what they can ask for is respect for the dignity and privacy of others (e.g., the essence of Mr. Y's roommate's complaint) or things like others' rights to have free access to public space and property (e.g., residents' complaints about the dining room table). Caregivers also may insist on Mrs. E's cooperation with her plan of care and should work toward resolving family members' concerns. But some would say that the private visits and public signs of affection should be beyond others' jurisdiction.

• Evaluating the role dementia plays: *What is the basis for restrictions?* Because of their vulnerability, persons with dementia need to be protected from harm. In addition, when there is loss of social inhibitions, others sometimes need to be protected from them. Harmful relationships between residents include those that involve exploitation (with or without harmful intent) and/or abuse. Discussing concerns about whether or not either party is at risk of being harmed or exploited is important. Surveillance provides evidence to support decisions about whether or not to restrict relationships. However, in situations similar to the example above, it may not always be clear when close surveillance could exceed individual rights to privacy, impose others' values, and constitute an affront to dignity. Surveillance also plays a role in protecting residents from being lost or hurt due to wandering or from being injured in falls and other accidents. It forms the basis of decisions about placing them on locked units to prevent them from leaving or judgments about use of physical and chemical restraints to prevent them from freely moving about. These decisions to restrict individuals' mobility tend to override their natural desires not to be restrained in favor of others' desires to ensure their safety.

• Consulting related sources: *How does one temper the culture of restrictive environments?* Federal regulations mandate respect for residents' dignity and their rights to self-determination, privacy, and freedom from any physical restraints or drugs, apart from those needed to treat medical symptoms. This requires nursing homes to reexamine protective care practices that rely on surveillance and restraint to control individuals. The way to temper a restrictive environment is to individualize care around these types of issues. There is much material to consult on restraint use (e.g., Castle et al., 1997; Dunbar et al., 1996; Evans et al., 1997; Sloane et al., 1991; Sullivan-

Marx, Strumpf, Evans, Baumgarten, & Maislin, 1999; Tinetti, Liu, Marottoli, & Ginter, 1991). And sources of information about intimacy, sexuality, and aging that can support discussions about appropriate and inappropriate sexual behavior, residents' sexual rights, and related policy development increasingly are available. For example, see Berger (2000), Kamel (2001), Miles & Parker (1999), Post (2000a), and Howe (2000) on sexuality and intimacy in the nursing home. Also, The Hebrew Home for the Aged at Riverdale, New York (2002a, 2002b) has developed a staff training manual ("Resident Sexuality in the Nursing Home") and video ("Freedom of Sexual Expression: Dementia and Resident Rights in Long-Term Care Facilities") with support from the New York State Department of Health Dementia Grants Program (distributor: Terra Nova Films). Topical references can help to guide thinking about what seems to make residents' lives worthwhile, how they communicate this information, and the basis for restricting persons from freely moving about, associating with others as they wish, and pursuing their rights without undue interference. In particular, caregivers need to reflect on resolutions made about persons with dementia. Are they being considered as individuals or does thinking about them follow prevailing stereotypes? Resources that shed light on the diversity and complexity of the resident population with diagnoses of dementia can help to maintain awareness that justifications for restriction or restraint should be based on the individual situation, not on blanket assumptions about what people with dementia are like.

Defining community norms and values involves people's positive moral rights, such as the right to attend community events, to have opportunities to form relationships, and to obtain a fair share of available goods, services, and amenities.

Example: Mr. G makes noisy gurgling, gagging sounds before spitting on the floor, or he spits into a kleenex, when reminded, and drops that on the floor. There also is a persistent smell of urine about him, his clothes, and his shoes because he denies that he is incontinent and refuses to wear protective briefs. His incontinence has been unresponsive to medical and behavioral interventions. And, although he reluctantly will yield to staff insistence that he bathe and change his clothes, it is difficult to completely eradicate the odor. Mr. G is alert, active, and very interested in all sorts of social activities. However, other residents do not want to be near him because of the way he smells, and no one wants to be his tablemate because of the spitting. (He has a private room.) There are periods of slight improve-

*ment whenever staff talk with him about the problem. But he does not
retain the information for very long. He continues to attend community
activities, despite other residents' complaints that he is too disgusting for
words and should be barred. Questions include: If insufficient memory
and cognitive awareness make it difficult for Mr. G to appropriately manage
these disturbing behaviors, what alternatives do staff have to improve the
situation? What are the infection control risks or issues? What responsibility
does the staff have to continue to support Mr. G's desires to be involved
in community life? What responsibility does the staff have to Mr. G's
disgruntled resident peers?*

Discussion about particular cases might involve:

• Examining institutional policies: *What do written policies about
residents' rights and residents' responsibilities say?* Residents have the right
to participate in community activities and to discuss issues and raise
complaints in Resident Council. Stated resident responsibilities generally include ideas about treating other residents with courtesy;
cooperating with staff in following their health care plan; assisting
staff in keeping the nursing home an attractive, safe, and healthy
place in which to live; and adhering to reasonable house rules
adopted for the health, safety, and comfort of the resident population
as a whole.

• Searching for meaning in residents' actions: *What do the resident's ideas about him/herself in relation to other residents seem to be?* The
above example does not explain Mr. G's motivation for attending
activities (e.g., interest in the activity and/or in being with other
people, something to do/relief from boredom or loneliness), nor
does it say anything about if and/or how he relates to other people.
The issue presents in terms of how the resident community responds
to him. But in pursuing an actual case, it would be important to
develop a portrait of Mr. G as an individual to promote understanding
of what he is seeking through his participation in community life. It
may or may not involve interest in relating to others. What he does
(e.g., ignores/engages with/antagonizes others) and what he seems
to experience (e.g., pleasure, discomfort, no reaction in response to
others) provide clues about his personal outlook. If alternative activities with more accepting individuals could be found for him, it would
be important to know what effect a change from the usual might
have. *What is the balance between individual and communal rights?* A
community's tolerance of particular individuals sometimes becomes

an issue in nursing homes. When intolerance involves misunderstanding or prejudice, discussion with involved individuals often works to restore balance. When a resident's loss of control over body, actions, or emotions is involved, how other residents' well-being is affected and what is fair to expect from them must be considered. Community norms and values influence the balance between maintaining individual rights with the least amount of intervention or restriction and maintaining communal rights with the greatest amount of fairness.

  • Evaluating the role dementia plays: *What kinds of community involvement are most beneficial for residents with dementia?* From an individual point of view, there is no uniform answer to this question. However, from an organizational point of view, it is important to consider the benefits of a multi-level targeted approach to providing opportunities to residents for community involvement. Facility-wide programming of activities is an effective approach for certain events (e.g., religious services, large-scale entertainment, picnics, and field trips); and, overall, it is more cost efficient. But, at the same time, reliance on one activity level, no matter how varied in content, places a portion of residents with dementia at a disadvantage. Obviously disadvantaged are individuals who become over-stimulated by being with too many people, persons with needs to wander about, those who overly disturb others and may need a companion, and persons who are afraid to leave the familiarity of their own living unit. Less obviously disadvantaged are passive attendees whose responses to life around them require more time to assess by facilitators of the activity who may not know them and do not have that kind of time. Facilities that move toward a balance with more unit-based/small group community activities built around residents' retained abilities and interests, with stable staff leaders who know the residents, and with allowances for one-on-one kinds of interaction, often find that even individuals with advanced dementia respond positively. *How should cognitively intact residents be encouraged to relate to residents with dementia?* The greater number of residents with dementia in a facility will not be on special care units. On the one hand, many persons will do well in the company of more cognitively intact residents, who in some cases may be very nurturing and provide good socialization. Facility staff generally work hard to make "good matches" of individuals they think will get along well together. On the other hand, it is not the responsibility of residents to care for peers, nor are well-meaning attentions of another resident always healthy for the person with dementia. Therefore, it is good not to take close helping relationships between residents for granted and to be sure that individuals are not being exploited or oppressed. Although they should not be encouraged to become "surrogate caregivers" and may need to be sheltered from others' disturbing behaviors, cognitively intact residents do have a responsibility to be "good neighbors" to those among them that may need more patience and understanding. Staff need to model desired behaviors so that residents can learn how to interact with one another. Furthermore, some residents are not kind, especially to persons with dementia. Ethical issues involving residents who mistreat others sometimes can be resolved, not only by staff setting a good example, but by staff kindly and continually insisting that being in a nursing home does not excuse them from being courteous and considerate.

  • Consulting related sources: *What activities promote and support a sense of community spirit?* There are many useful resources that suggest types of activities that may be used to engage nursing home residents, some focused on those with dementia. Planned activities are tools that can be used effectively or ineffectively. But they cannot, in themselves, promote community spirit. The spirit of any community is in relationships that exist among its membership. Residents, families, and staff are the core members of nursing home communities. Following are examples of unscheduled activities that each component of the core can perform to promote and support a sense of community spirit. Persons smile and greet each other as they pass. Thanks and compliments are exchanged regularly. Life's joys and sorrows are acknowledged and shared. Communication is spontaneous and inclusive. In nursing homes where these activities occur with some frequency, residents know that they are loved, families know that they are members of the team, staff know that they are valued, and everyone knows that they are appreciated. These are qualities of relationships that are not easily measured and can never be exercised to perfection. But in their absence, the spirit of a community suffers. It is never too early or too late to note the essence of community relationships and to consider its moral impact on the meaningfulness and effectiveness of planned/unplanned activities.

DIMENSIONS OF THE TAXONOMY

Positive and Negative Moral Rights

Positive and negative moral rights both involve duties. But duties to uphold a person's negative rights (e.g., not to be forced, restrained, confined, or intruded upon) may be comparatively simpler to describe and carry out. In contrast, upholding a person's positive rights (e.g., to do as one wishes, attend community events, have opportunities to form relationships, and obtain a fair share of available goods, services, and amenities) might be complicated by others' competing claims (issues of fairness and personal consideration) and decisions about the use of limited resources. Therefore, an approach to ethics case analysis needs to be able to deal with resident-focused issues in ways that do not lose sight of the various ramifications for other individuals and for the nursing home community as a whole. The following steps may be useful in moving this taxonomic conceptualization of the issues into a process format for conducting a case analysis.

Case Analysis

Clinical ethics is a form of applied ethics historically oriented toward cases arising in hospital settings. A classic example is Jonsen, Siegler, and Winslade's (1998) approach to ethical decisions in clinical medicine. Although different in organizational format, the described use of the taxonomy has much in common with what these authors hold to be important aspects of case analysis: (a) medical indications; (b) patient preferences; (c) quality of life; and (d) contextual features. In adapting their clinical ethics model to a long-term care/nursing home focus, for purposes of discussion, the term "medical indications" has been changed to "ethical issues"; and the term "patient preferences" has been changed to "resident preferences."

Ethical Issues

What are the resident-related concerns? Who is affected by these concerns? What is the resident's physical, social, and emotional condition? What is the plan of care? How is the plan of care expected to benefit and avoid harm to the resident?

In the clinical ethics model, discussion focuses first on the patient's pathological condition and indications for medical treatment/intervention, including the immediate benefits to be gained versus any risks. This treatment of disease focus is too narrow for nursing homes. However, cases still need to unfold with a description of concerns, the resident's condition, and rationales underlying his/her care plan and service needs.

The first step in case analysis is to conceptualize the issues that constitute the ethical concern. The above taxonomy is like a wheel.

Everyday concerns affecting residents' lives revolve around its inter-secting planes (defined in terms of individual and social values) and may, at different times, be illuminated by one or another of its four domains. But the domains cannot be separated from the whole. There-fore, choosing to use the focus of one domain to draw out the ethical nature of an issue does not diminish the relevance of them all to a resident's situation. However, for awhile, this focus may encourage the facts of the case to emerge.

The facts of the case may be the familiar types of concerns that are routinely addressed in a value-neutral way (i.e., there are general procedures and clinical protocols that practitioners can use to deal with any of the issues that have been discussed above). However, the ethical elements embedded in these situations are brought forward when the same concerns are framed in a value-laden manner (i.e., issues of rights, duties, and principles). The facts remain the same. The situation first needs to be described in detail. Then the process becomes one of question-discovery.

Resident Preferences

What preferences has the resident expressed? Has the resident expressed prior preferences (e.g., advance directives)? Who is the resident's designated surrogate? Has the resident/family been informed of the resident's rights, responsibilities, and plan of care? What is the resident's decisional capacity/legal competency? Is the resident's right to choice and self-determination being respected, ethically and legally?

The ethical principle that directs attention to resident preferences is respect for autonomy, the moral right to self-determination and freedom of choice. There are several ways in which resident preferences may be known. The first way is to listen to what residents say and to ask them directly. This may seem simplistic, but to listen and to ask in a truly attentive way requires effort and understanding. With all persons, and especially those with dementia, the gift of unhurried time is im-portant. Persons with cognition and language difficulties cannot always find the right words to express their wishes, particularly when they are under pressure of time to do so. Getting to know a person through time spent with him/her in quiet moments is the basis for validating and correcting one's assumptions about the individual's preferences against his/her own reality as it comes to be understood through the formation of a relationship.

A second way to deduce a resident's preferences is through direct observation. Some family caregivers can provide helpful interpretations based on their experiences. And certified nursing assistants who care regularly for the person become expert at reading his/her mood and observing signs that others would miss or misinterpret. They come to know intuitively what the resident's preferences are and, therefore, often are able to adjust their approaches to care accordingly. This knowledge needs to be shared.

A third way to clarify or intuit resident preferences requires the use of prior knowledge of the person and his/her wishes. Ideally, the substituted judgment of a surrogate or proxy is based on prior knowledge of the resident, but staff seldom know residents apart from the institutional setting. What makes residents unique can be lost in institutional record keeping that increasingly comes to reflect how they are and what they do in the context of the nursing home. In this way, residents' individuality can become less connected with their own past and more directed toward comparing them with their institutionalized peers. Thus, intuiting what residents' preferences might be must get beyond limited institutional representations that do not do them justice to an informed understanding of the qualities that characterized persons pre-institutionally.

The principles of autonomy and beneficence (doing good and putting others' interests first) conflict when others act in the "best interests" of residents who lack decisional capacity or competence. Whether or not this constitutes paternalism (control that challenges/undermines personal autonomy) is a question that always should be asked when it occurs in cases where preferences are not known and, especially, in cases when resident preferences are ignored or overruled. If acting in another's "best interests" (beneficence) is judged to be the greater good, overriding autonomy may be justified. But paternalism, as it generally has come to be understood in clinical ethics, is not acceptable.

Quality of Life

How does the resident view his/her quality of life? How do persons other than the resident view his/her quality of life? How is the plan of care expected to improve or maintain the resident's quality of life? Are there any plans to forego treatment? What plans are in place for comfort/palliative care?

In clinical ethics, discussions involving the estimated quality of a person's life concern the long-term consequences of continuing, foregoing, or rationing care. Jonsen et al. (1998) point out that all conversations about medical treatment are about quality of life, despite the fact that the definition of this concept is vague. Thus, enhancing quality of life through, for example, relief of pain (including palliative/comfort

care to the dying) would be cause to initiate or continue certain therapies. But care that has no benefits or has undesirable effects that out-
weigh limited benefits will raise questions about foregoing treatment.
And, when quality of life falls below what these authors call "lower than
minimal" (e.g., when resuscitation or life support cannot reverse a
persistent deteriorating physical process or when death seems imminent), the discussion turns to withholding or discontinuing treatment.
Deliberation also may be complicated by decisions involving the use of
limited or expensive resources (e.g., costly drugs or hemodialysis) that
raise questions about who should benefit. In the face of scarcity and
expense, issues of rationing or bias (i.e., beliefs about how treatments
might benefit one person more or less than other persons in various
circumstances) may influence decisions.

Nursing homes have their share of cases where ethical analysis involves decisions about initiating, continuing, or withholding treatment.
Because the population largely is composed of frail individuals with
multiple chronic medical conditions, there always will be occasion to
weigh the merits of clinically intervening to maintain or enhance quality
of life as it pertains to treating disease and alleviating associated physi-
cal/mental distress. Here, the resident's wishes and best interests are
intertwined with family wishes and staff concerns, giving rise to various
ethical issues. For example, lack of agreement among residents, family,
and staff on what should be done in a specific instance will need to be
resolved. Lack of clarity about resident wishes, when residents can no
longer express their views about the quality of life they would like to
have, as well as discomfort of surrogates and others in carrying out
residents' advance directives, require careful deliberation. And it is
equally important to determine the extent to which ageism is involved
in negative assumptions about frail elderly people's quality of life that
are used as reasons to deny them more expensive, less readily available
forms of care.

Nursing homes also have broader issues related to residents' quality
of life that extend beyond clinical treatment concerns. For example,
quality of life (QOL) is related to residents' personal and social needs
to find meaningfulness in their daily pursuits, to experience happiness,
and to participate in satisfying relationships. But only the resident knows
what, specifically, makes his/her life meaningful, enjoyable, and satisfying. When dementia diminishes an individual's ability to comprehend
and to communicate such subjective thoughts in words, ways need
to be found to understand what responses to others and to his/her
environment may indicate about perceived QOL. Volumes edited by
Volicer and Bloom-Charette (1999) and by Albert and Logsdon (2000)

on QOL in persons with dementia present good introductions to the multiple ethical and practical issues of developing appropriate measures and interventions to better understand and care for individuals who have varying degrees of cognitive impairment. In the latter volume, Jennings (2000) suggests that respect for moral personhood is the ethical basis for pursuing what QOL in dementia care means.

> It is one thing to give care and protection out of a sense of pity, or charity, or professional duty, or even love; it is another to maintain relationship and connection with the other for as long as possible out of a sense of the moral importance of that connection per se. Caring and caregiving, after all, are not only about meeting an individual's needs or making him comfortable; they are about the recognition of the person of the other, the one being cared for, and they are about the caregiver's own personhood therein also. I have just said the recognition of the person of the other; I should also say that caregiving and quality of life are about the preserving, conserving, sustaining, nurturing, and eliciting of that personhood as well. (p. 175)

Contextual Features

What resident-related factors (e.g., personal history; social, economic, religious, cultural variables) may influence recommendations? What institutional factors (e.g., allocation of resources, staffing, work patterns, policies, administration, physical/social environment) may influence recommendations?

Understanding the contexts within which all cases are embedded is essential to their resolution. Residents come from diverse backgrounds and have different lifestyles with many types of social network relationships. Network members, particularly families and close friends, may express interest and play important roles. They often provide emotional and material support to the resident and are a good source of information and advice about his/her life and values. They also may raise concerns about the resident's care and question decisions in both helpful and controversial ways. When resident and family member relationships are strained or problematic, staff can be caught in the history of these past entanglements. At other times, family members or surrogates may seem to be seeking to serve their own needs or interests before those of the resident. The roles of relatives and friends need to be understood so that their cooperation can be engaged in service of the resident's needs. At the same time, their needs for comfort and support often are very great. Thus, ethical resolution of a resident's concerns also needs to be directed toward understanding and caring for significant persons in his/her life.

The restrictive homogenizing nature of institutional environments will be the cause of some ethical concerns, and organizational policies and practices will be the cause of others. The nursing home experience itself (Chapter 2) is the context within which resident issues and concerns need to be understood. Many residents and families come reluctantly, having exhausted all other possibilities (Chapter 1). Therefore, their concerns first must be understood within the context of whatever symbolic meaning the nursing home transition has for them (e.g., symbol of loss for residents/guilt for families; a major turning point symbolizing the resident's decline/foreshadowing death; a haven or refuge symbolizing safety and relief). For many, the rigors of communal life are a challenge; and interpersonal relationships with staff and other residents are new and different (Chapters 2 and 3). Thus, concerns also must be understood within the context of the practical realities that encompass their everyday lives (e.g., institutional schedules and service patterns; policies; care provider work assignments; room-sharing and other environmental features; activities; patterns of social interaction). Much of the preceding discussion has been about this kind of context (i.e., nursing home culture). Finally, it is good to acknowledge and develop an understanding of the community/public contexts (e.g., local, state, and national) that influence nursing home policies and practices. Although this book focuses on micro-level issues (i.e., resident cases) rather than on these broader contexts, awareness of macro-level regulatory and public policy issues can lend added perspective to individual case analysis.

In summary, in Jonsen et al.'s (1998) clinical ethics model, *contextual features* help to make sense and bring together the details of a case that are drawn out by description of the *ethical issues, resident preferences,* and *quality of life* considerations. The authors describe it as an effort to orient the case analysis process to the realities that practitioners encounter in clinical settings.

> Many books on health care ethics are organized around moral principles, such as respect for autonomy, beneficence, nonmaleficence, and fairness, and the cases are analyzed in the light of those principles. Our method is different. While we appreciate the importance of principles . . . the authors believe that clinicians need a straightforward way to sort the facts and values of the case at hand into an orderly pattern that will facilitate the discussion and resolution of the ethical problem. (Jonsen et al., 1998, p. 2)

In similar fashion, an approach can be patterned around the taxonomy to facilitate discussion and resolution of everyday ethical issues. It involves identifying a domain that best illustrates the issue and illuminating resident preferences, quality of life concerns, and contextual features in the process of bringing together the facts of the case. This process may be aided by addressing the following previously illustrated four areas.

Examining institutional policies provides understanding of the nursing home's formal written position on the topic or, in some cases, the unwritten practices that cause the organization to function as it does. *Searching for meaning in residents' actions* demonstrates respect for the individual and his/her efforts to communicate a distinct point of view. *Evaluating the role dementia plays* assumes knowledge of what dementia is and how it affects person's lives that goes beyond surface assumptions and stereotypes. And *consulting related sources* provides insight and support for recommendations based on credible materials produced outside of the localized nursing home situation. Useful reference materials are being produced continually, and it is best to hand-select what may be most up-to-date or relevant to the situation under discussion when that time is at hand.

CASE PRESENTATION

The sample cases that follow illustrate the use of the taxonomy. However, this does not preclude blending the two frameworks, as illustrated in the discussion about ethics committee functions in the appendix. Here it is shown how Jonsen et al.'s (1998) organizing strategy could serve as a vehicle for the taxonomy. Thus, what really matters is that ethics committees discover the formats that serve them best, which may include those of their own invention.

The sample cases that follow in this book are examples of characteristic ethical concerns that could apply to everyday experiences in any nursing home. They tell a partial story and invite the reader to imagine what might, from an ethical point of view, be a fitting ending. But they do not provide as much detailed information as an actual case might, thus creating the opportunity for readers to identify what additional questions about the hypothetical resident's situation would need to be raised and answered.

Formal presentation of an actual case could, in a more detailed fashion, follow this pattern of a single integrated descriptive account. Another presentational style might use a descriptive approach that breaks out different types of information and points of view, (e.g., sections for resident concerns, medical history, psychosocial background, nursing perspective, pastoral care summary, family perspective, etc.). Written presentation of the case description then could be fol-

lowed by discussion questions and resource reading designed to support
dialogue about the ethical issues that leads to recommendations and a
possible resolution.

ANALYTIC STYLES

These *descriptive* semi-structured formats lend themselves to different
styles of ethical analysis. For example, *ethical principles and moral values*
can come into play through the process of thinking about and discussing
a case.

> Sometimes cases involve "competing goods"—e.g., (and with reference to
> above case examples): It is good to have the right to refuse care (*autonomy*)
> vs. it is good to provide necessary care (*beneficence/non-maleficence*) . . . It is
> good to follow the resident's advance directives (*autonomy/fidelity*) vs. it is
> good to use treatment to increase comfort or relieve pain (*beneficence*) . . . It
> is good to organize care around the resident's wishes (*autonomy*) vs. it is good
> to organize care around what benefits the greatest number of residents (*justice
> or fairness*) . . . It is good to support *individual values* and needs for intimacy
> vs. it is good to respect *community values* and needs regarding expressions of
> intimacy . . . It is good to support individual wishes and privileges to attend
> group activities (*autonomy/individual justice*) vs. it is good to be honest with the
> individual and others about unacceptable social behaviors (*veracity/ fairness*).
> Other cases may invite debate over whether specific actions made in the
> person's best interests (*beneficence*) constitute a greater moral good or are
> examples of paternalism. Or they may focus on how residents with dementia
> express *autonomy*.

A casuistic analytic style will lay out the facts of the case, inviting
comparisons to determine what was helpful in other similar cases as
well as what is unique about the case under discussion (i.e., its differences and nuances). But, although it may seek paradigm examples to
illuminate moral principles and values, it leans away from rule-based
ideas about treating everyone the same way. Thus, each case rests on
its own merits. Similarly, *narrative analysis* focuses on laying out the facts
of a case. But it uses individual case description as a dramatic vehicle
to explore the meanings a situation may have for a person based on
his/her life story and, from that point of view, to project what an
appropriate resolution of the case might be.

The variety and abundance of ethical issues affecting nursing home
residents with dementia will come as no surprise to persons familiar
with nursing homes. Descriptions here only touch upon some that are
encountered daily. Additionally, in these settings multiple workplace

demands vie for the time and attention of nursing home personnel who share responsibility for ethical resolution of issues and concerns. It is with these assumptions in mind that an appendix, following the sample cases and commentaries in Chapter 4, extends the above focus on case presentation and analysis to a discussion of nursing home ethics committees.

4

Case Examples

OVERVIEW

This chapter provides 12 hypothetical case examples of resident-focused situations illustrating a range of ordinary concerns that have ethical implications. The narratives are fictitious and do not represent actual persons or events. However, the situations and ethical issues are drawn from true experiences of multiple nursing home residents, family, and staff members. The examples were designed for use in nursing homes as practice cases for ethics committees or as staff in-service education offerings. The intent is to simulate a review of ethical issues that may yield a variety of perspectives and perhaps more than one recommended action. Readers can use the dialogue-commentary format as a self-paced exercise or the materials can be used with a group. In-service education instructors may wish to know about the readability measures performed on the case narratives with Word software Grammar Check. Each readability score bases its rating on the average number of syllables per word and words per sentence.

Flesch-Kincaid Grade Level Score = 8.7
This measure rates text on a U.S. grade-school level, for example, a score of 8.0 means that an 8th grader can understand the document. For most standard documents, a 7th or 8th grade reading level is recommended.

Flesch Reading Ease Score = 62
This measure rates text on a 100-point scale. The higher the score, the easier it is to understand the document. The recommended score for most standard documents is one of approximately 60–70.

After each case narrative there is a section called *Dialogue* in which "questions" and "possible actions" (i.e., ways in which individuals might respond) are presented as beginning ideas to stimulate thoughtfulness and discussion. Readers/participants may have additional ideas based on their own experiences. The earlier introduced taxonomy is used to focus issues and suggest directions that might be taken in pursuing each case: examining institutional policies; searching for meaning in residents' actions; evaluating the role dementia plays; and consulting related sources. The *Commentary* section simulates dialogue about possible actions. "Possible actions" are not necessarily "right" or "wrong," but it could be argued that some may be better than others. The aim is not to close down conversation but, rather, to leave it open to different ideas and interpretations. (In actual cases, examination of the ethical issues would permit more detailed discussion about a known resident's preferences, quality of life considerations, and contextual features of the specific situation.)

Use of the dialogue and commentary sections can be flexible. For example, all "possible actions" may be ranked or evaluated for what are judged to be the best responses. Another approach would be to have members of a group discuss a case example among themselves and recommend other courses of action, before commenting on the prepared list of possible responses to the issue. Groups also might want to engage in role-playing.

(The reader will notice that both given and surnames are used in the following narratives, calling attention to how forms of address vary. This is a serious ethical issue. The position here is that, to be respectful and avoid causing offense, proper titles—Mr., Mrs., Miss, Dr., Rev.—and surnames should be used to address residents. A given name or nickname should be used only if that is what the resident prefers. Some would say that no resident should be addressed by a given name. Others favor resident's choice. But what is never acceptable is assuming that it is all right to call an adult by his/her given name without being requested or given permission to do so.)

CASE EXAMPLE 1. MY FAVORITE THINGS

Ruby Pierce is an 82-year-old widow who has lived at Evergreen Manor for almost one year. She left her home in a distant city at the urging of her son, who had been observing a decline in his mother's ability to manage her own affairs. Her family visits regularly, and Mrs. Pierce has made an effort to settle into her new life by becoming an enthusiastic participant in a variety of social activities. She knows her way around Friendship Place (the name of her residential unit), having quickly established a personal routine and a circle of friends and acquaintances with whom she easily passes the time. She also likes to sit quietly by herself after the evening meal and crochet items that she often gives to others as gifts.

Though Mrs. Pierce has a number of chronic conditions, including diabetes, heart disease, and arthritis, she is medically stable and independent in self care. She enjoys selecting just the right pieces of jewelry to go with an impressive collection of elegant suits and dresses and she takes time to be assured that her makeup and hair style are exactly right before venturing outside her room. The diagnosis of beginning stage Alzheimer's disease, which accounted for her need to move to a more protective environment, has not impeded her ability to socialize and interact with others. However, in the past few months she has become increasingly forgetful and now needs regular prompting when it is time for the activities that she especially enjoys. "I just seem to lose track of time," she explains, and she is acutely disappointed when activities are missed for lack of someone reminding or coming to get her. "My days and weeks are all in a muddle," she says with regard to her schedule. "But, you know, what really bothers me the most is that I have been missing some of my favorite things . . . things that are very precious to me. Someone has taken them, and I wish I knew who it was because I'm sure those little articles could never mean so much to anyone else as they do to me." Missing items (such as jewelry, glasses, crochet hooks, makeup, shoes, and sweaters) sometimes have been found in Mrs. Pierce's room—in the back of the closet, at the bottom of drawers, in the wastebasket, and under the mattress. A crochet hook also was found under a chair cushion in a small sitting room to which Mrs. Pierce retires in the evening to work on her projects.

Other residents on Mrs. Pierce's floor are becoming agitated and alarmed about the potential threat to their possessions, as they hear her accounts of lost articles on a daily basis. She has persuaded them that the keys they all have to secure items in top dresser drawers pose little safeguard to the danger of rampant theft. They, in turn, have accounts of their own experiences with missing items, though none as recent or persistent as Mrs. Pierce's. Concerns about the safety of personal property have been raised in Resident Council meetings, and gossip among residents is full of speculation about which residents or staff members are most suspect or least trustworthy in the court of popular opinion.

Mrs. Pierce's son is concerned about his mother's complaints and has asked to review institutional policies and procedures related to missing property. He has asked to see reports filed on each missing item and has inquired about the process used to document what has been found and to locate the whereabouts of lost articles. In light of evidence suggesting that Mrs. Pierce herself may be responsible for misplacing things, he is open to staff member opinions that the situation may reflect her struggles with progressive dementia. However, he is ambivalent in the face of his mother's emphatic and articulate assessment of the situation and his own opinion that theft is a real problem in even the best nursing homes. He wants to be supportive of nursing home staff, with whom he is generally satisfied, but his loyalty as a good son is to his mother.

Nursing and housekeeping staff members on Mrs. Pierce's floor are weary and dispirited with the barrage of innuendoes and accusations that they feel are being leveled against them. They are convinced that Mrs. Pierce misplaces and hides the items she later accuses others (generally staff members) of stealing. And although they acknowledge that this may be a manifestation of her disease, as one staff member put it, "It still feels bad; and you still have to find a way to work with her, all the time knowing she may be thinking and saying nasty untrue things about you." Additionally, staffs from other disciplines, such as recreation and social service, have found it difficult to keep organized activities on track because Mrs. Pierce's long and repetitious stories about her missing items have become a major obstruction to programs. Moreover, her needs to express grief and concern threaten to overshadow other residents' needs to participate in their own ways. When attention is refocused on the matter at hand or Mrs. Pierce is asked to relinquish the floor so that another resident may have a turn to speak, she falls into tearful silence, which effectively puts a damper on others' enjoyment of the scheduled event.

POSITIVE RIGHT: PRESERVING INDIVIDUAL INTEGRITY

The immediate issue is one of respect for Mrs. Pierce's dignity and the meaning her possessions have for her. The needs and rights of other residents and staff also are a consideration. Respect for personal property is the larger organizational-level issue.

Dialogue

Where is the *ethical conflict* or dilemma of *competing goods*?

Are there *questions* brought to mind but not answered by the narrative?

Institutional policies: What are the policies on care and safeguarding of residents' personal property? What are the options for residents to be able to lock up valuables or to lock the doors of private rooms? What is done to prevent other residents who have difficulty recognizing what does and does not belong to them from taking or disturbing other residents' property? Is there an active theft prevention program? What procedures are followed in reporting and following up on missing items? What is the recovery rate for lost property?

Meaning in resident's actions: In what ways do Mrs. Pierce's possessions help to define who she is as an individual? Why are her belongings important to her?

The role dementia plays: How does dementia affect some persons' ability to care for and keep track of personal property and to distinguish their possessions from those of others? Why might Mrs. Pierce believe that her belongings have been stolen? What if some of her things have been stolen? If no one believes her, will she be more vulnerable to theft?

Related sources: Harris & Benson (2000). Theft in nursing homes; Powers (in press) The significance of losing things for nursing home residents with dementia and their families.

What are pros and cons of the following *possible actions*? Are there *other recommendations*?

Possible Actions:

1. Move Mrs. Pierce to avoid disruption of social events and preserve peace for the greater number of residents, whom she seems to be upsetting. On a unit with more cognitively compromised residents, she may produce a less unsettling effect overall.

2. Suggest that the son take some jewelry and other items home with him, leaving a more limited number of things to monitor. This would be followed by the creation of a personal property checklist and a strategy, to be worked out with Mrs. Pierce, to identify clearly designated places for each article on the checklist.

3. Review institutional policies and procedures related to safeguarding residents' personal property and involve staff in discussions about zero tolerance for theft, dealing with hurt when unjustly accused, and addressing issues of missing property with residents and their families.

4. Suggest that Mrs. Pierce's son prepare a handwritten list of valued items and have him tape record himself reassuring her not to worry . . . that all her belongings are safe. Reaffirming the presence of each item, with the help of staff and the list in her son's handwriting, as well as listening to his familiar voice on the tape

may decrease Mrs. Pierce's general anxiety about the safety and whereabouts of her possessions.

5. Prepare an attractive container to serve as Mrs. Pierce's "treasure chest" and encourage her to keep her most precious belongings in it.

6. When confronted by Mrs. Pierce over a missing object, suggest enthusiastically—"Why don't we go and look for it?" Start immediately, following up on hunches (e.g., "Let's look in the family room?" "Were you in the craft room today?") and accompanying her on an active search.

7. Have a lost and found area (e.g., a large drawer or a set of shelves) where residents, families, or staff members know they may leave or retrieve misplaced items.

8. Provide a private room that can be locked by Mrs. Pierce with a key she can keep on a wrist holder. This would limit access to her room by other residents and persons not entrusted with the master key.

Commentary on My Favorite Things

Ethical Considerations

Ethical principles of doing good (beneficence) and being fair (justice) are involved. Considerate and respectful care of Mrs. Pierce includes listening to and not dismissing her concerns. Being fair to others involves considering the feelings and needs of unit staff and other residents.

Competing Goods Might Be:

It is good to respect Mrs. Pierce's concerns about her missing property.

It is good to respect the sensitivity of staff members who may be wrongly accused.

It is good to listen to Mrs. Pierce every time she relates this concern.

It is good to allow comparable opportunities for other residents to express themselves.

It is good to be flexible in managing organized activities to allow for the unexpected.

It is good to be on track with organized activities for the sake of the larger audience.

Questions

We do not know other residents' views of Mrs. Pierce as a person. When she monopolizes conversation with repeated stories of her losses, are there objections from other residents? How do they respond to her? Might commiserating with her serve some purpose?

Is Mrs. Pierce encouraged to share with others the significance of some of her things that are not missing, allowing her to focus on valued possessions in a positive, self-affirming way?

Is Mrs. Pierce in a private room? If so, does she have the option of locking the door?

Discussion of *pros and cons of "possible actions"* might be as follows:

Possible Action #1

Move Mrs. Pierce to avoid disruption of social events and preserve peace for the greater number of residents, whom she seems to be upsetting. On a unit with more cognitively compromised residents, she may produce a less unsettling effect overall.

PRO: A different setting may minimize the effects of Mrs. Pierce's behavior on others.
CON: This action does not appear to be in the best interests of Mrs. Pierce. She seems to have made a comfortable adjustment to nursing home life on a unit where she knows her way around, has established friendships with other residents, and has a social life that complements her personal routines. Also, though other residents may be expressing concerns about the safety of their possessions, there is no evidence that Mrs. Pierce upsets them. She might be missed by her friends if she were to be moved, and having to make new friends with people who are more cognitively compromised than the people she knows could have a devastating effect on her.

Possible Action #2

Suggest that the son take some jewelry and other items home with him, leaving a more limited number of things to monitor. This would be followed by the creation of a personal property checklist and a strategy, to be worked out with Mrs. Pierce, to identify clearly designated places for each article on the checklist.

PRO: The success of this action depends on consensus regarding what stays and what goes. Mrs. Pierce and her son might reach an agreement about this.

CON: If agreement cannot be reached, the stage might be set for further upset because Mrs. Pierce may not want to part with her possessions. If she agrees to have her son take some for safekeeping, she may not remember later and believe that they are lost or stolen. And she may not be able to remember agreed upon designated places for items or be able to understand the concept of a checklist. In summary, this is a rational solution for an issue that might not lend itself to a logically reasoned approach.

Possible Action #3

Review institutional policies and procedures related to safeguarding residents' personal property and involve staff in discussions about zero tolerance for theft, dealing with hurt when unjustly accused, and addressing issues of missing property with residents and their families.

PRO: These actions are important. They imply that concerns like those of Mrs. Pierce and her son will be taken seriously and acted upon. Staff members also need to be reminded about what the consequences are for nursing home personnel who steal. But, at the same time, their feelings about being unjustly blamed or suspected of wrongdoing need to be acknowledged with time set aside to relieve stress and provide support. It is important to talk about how the situation makes staff feel. Hurt feelings may affect their relationships with Mrs. Pierce and her son and their willingness to sympathize and assist her in her distress. It also is a good time to review and reevaluate policies.

CON: This is not a comfortable topic.

Possible Action #4

Suggest that Mrs. Pierce's son prepare a handwritten list of valued items and have him tape record himself reassuring her not to worry . . . that all her belongings are safe. Reaffirming the presence of each item, with the help of staff and the list in her son's handwriting, as well as listening to his familiar voice on the tape may decrease Mrs. Pierce's general anxiety about the safety and whereabouts of her possessions.

PRO: This is a creative solution that has two strengths. First, the responsibility for monitoring items deemed valuable is shifted from Mrs. Pierce to her son in collaboration with unit staff. Second, the son's handwriting and voice on tape could have a reassuring and calming effect as long as Mrs. Pierce is able to trust that he and the staff have the matter under control.

CON: The limited usefulness of this action will surface when items go missing and cannot be found. And reassuring Mrs. Pierce that all is well when things are missing would be untruthful. Also, Mrs. Pierce may not respond positively to a tape recorded message or be able to understand its intended purpose. If she is not familiar with communicating with family in this fashion, it may frighten her.

Possible Action #5

Prepare an attractive container to serve as Mrs. Pierce's "treasure chest"; and encourage her to keep her most precious belongings in it.

PRO: This also is a creative solution. Its strength lies in the recognition that Mrs. Pierce's things are treasured, and it provides one obvious and attractive storage space for them in contrast to many undistinguishable, ordinary spaces (drawers, closets, etc.).

CON: The limited usefulness of this action will reveal itself at some point when an item is not returned to the "treasure chest" and cannot be found. Also, Mrs. Pierce may not be able to understand this procedure and use it.

Possible Action #6

When confronted by Mrs. Pierce over a missing object, suggest enthusiastically—"Why don't we go and look for it?" Start immediately, following up on hunches (e.g., "Let's look in the family room." "Were you in the craft room today?") and accompanying her on an active search.

PRO: This is a good choice because there is willingness to accept Mrs. Pierce's reality and join in an activity of some importance to her—trying to locate her missing items. Whether they are found or not, she may be comforted and have her spirits raised by this simple caring act.

CON: This will place greater time demands on staff members. Also, Mrs. Pierce may feel that staff are dismissing her belief that others have taken things and perceive that this approach implies that it is her fault.

Possible Action #7

Have a lost and found area (e.g., a large drawer or a set of shelves) where residents, families, or staff members know that they may leave or retrieve misplaced items.

PRO: This is not a bad idea. It creates a new place to look for Mrs. Pierce's missing items.

CON: But it also is an impersonal pragmatic arrangement that does not bring the individual needs of Mrs. Pierce into focus. What is needed is a personalized approach that will take her individual situation more into account.

Possible Action #8

Provide a private room that can be locked by Mrs. Pierce with a key she can keep on a wrist holder. This would limit access to her room by other residents and persons not entrusted with the master key.

PRO: Fewer persons would have access to Mrs. Pierce's belongings. Other residents would not be a source of concern. And Mrs. Pierce might experience a greater sense of reassurance over ability to exercise more control and oversight.

CON: If property is missing, Mrs. Pierce may voice new worries about who may have a key to her room. Or she might lose the key.

CASE EXAMPLE 2. BREAKING BAD NEWS

Steve Henning is a 78-year-old man whose wife moved in with him when he came to live at New Life Nursing Home five years ago. The first year they shared a room on a floor for residents whose needs for supervision and assistance with personal care were minimal. Mr. Henning's physical health was good, but his progressive dementia caused him to be increasingly forgetful and confused. He willingly accepted direction from Mildred, his wife of many years, whose physical health was declining as a result of chronic obstructive pulmonary disease with cardiac complications. Mildred was impatient with Steve. She screamed and talked rudely to him when he didn't follow her instructions. Steve just smiled pleasantly and allowed her to order him about. In contrast to this pleasing behavior with his wife, though, Steve was becoming increasingly antagonistic toward other residents' efforts to protect themselves from his intrusions. He walked and wandered in and out of their rooms, sometimes disturbing their belongings or lying down on their beds. When asked to leave, he often became upset and angry. Mildred could neither keep up with him nor keep him sufficiently occupied. She reluctantly agreed to Steve's transfer to the special care unit where his behavior might be better tolerated, while she remained behind in a smaller private room.

Staff members observed that for months each seemed lost without the other. They had been married for 55 years and rarely had been separated. At first Mildred would come up on the elevator by herself to visit Steve. However, the behavior of other residents on the floor irritated her, and when she began to slap and yell at them too, it was decided that it would be better to have staff bring Steve downstairs to visit with her. Every day Mildred would be waiting eagerly at the elevator for Steve. They ate noon and evening meals together in the dining room on her floor and Mildred would ask the unit secretary to call and have her husband brought down to accompany her to events and activities as well. No one doubted Mildred's devotion to Steve, despite her belligerent and bossy ways with him. Indeed, her frustration seemed to grow as her health failed and his ability to understand and comply with her wishes similarly decreased. After an hour or two of being yelled at and shoved around by Mildred, staff thought Steve seemed relieved to be returned to his floor. In time, staff began to wonder if his resistance when they mentioned getting ready to go see Mildred was his way of communicating that he did not want to be subjected to any more of her rough treatment. But they could only speculate because Steve often was resistant to their own efforts to assist with his personal care.

Children, grandchildren, and nieces and nephews frequently visited Steve and Mildred and reinforced an understanding of the two as a loving couple from a tight-knit family. Together they had worked long hours in a small business which they owned and operated and they enjoyed parties, dancing, and socializing with relatives and friends. They were described as "lovebirds," always kissing, holding hands, and openly expressing affection for one another. Family members felt especially sorry for Steve, whose abilities to communicate and to indicate whether or not he understood who people were or what they were saying to him became seriously compromised. At the same time they excused Mildred's frustrated outbursts at him, declaring her a saint for battling on against the relentless grasp of his severe and worsening dementia.

New behavior for Steve included short periods of time in the late morning or early afternoon, when he would cry, wail, and give an occasional pound on the wall with his fist as he paced. He responded well to a calm presence on the part of any staff member walking along beside him, listening and murmuring gently in response to a torrent of incoherent speech that erupted from him at these times. Physically exhausted, he would eventually allow himself to be led to a chair or his bed to rest. Later he would appear to be cheerful and no worse from these episodes. However, the episodes of upset behavior sometimes coincided with the times Steve was wanted downstairs by Mildred. It was difficult for her to accept that he was unable to leave the floor when he was in one of these states. More than ever she wanted to see what she could do to soothe him. But she was unsuccessful when she came up to see him and tried.

Visits between Mildred and Steve became less routine, although she asked about him daily. Steve gave no sign of recognizing her when they were together and he became more quiet and passive in the interim between emotional upsets. As he began to establish a daily routine of his own, he appeared to become fearful of leaving his floor. Offers to take him to see Mildred or to bring Mildred up to see him brought forth no response. When Mildred became acutely ill, staff or family took him down briefly and stayed with the couple in her room. This was seen as more of a benefit for Mildred, who would reach out to touch Steve, hold his hand, and ask earnestly about his health and well being. Steve responded by becoming very still and withdrawn.

Early one morning, Mildred died quietly in her sleep. Family members were notified, and two sons and their families spent time with Steve telling him about Mildred's death and about arrangements for her funeral. They told the chaplain and the head nurse that they could detect no sign that their father was aware of what had happened and they were divided in their opinions about whether any further effort should be made to relay the potentially upsetting information. Staff members also are not in agreement over talking with Steve about his loss. Consequently, there is an air of uncertainty with nobody immediately taking a strong stand with regard to the question: Should anything or should nothing more be done to break the bad news?

POSITIVE RIGHT: PRESERVING INDIVIDUAL INTEGRITY

The issue is one of respect and compassion for an individual who has suffered a personal loss. The effect of Mildred's death on other residents and staff also needs to be considered. The ways in which significant life events are recognized is the larger organizational issue.

Dialogue

Where is the *ethical conflict* or dilemma of *competing goods*?

Are there *questions* brought to mind but not answered by the narrative?

Institutional policies: What are policies and practices related to informing families, residents, and staff about deaths of loved ones and/or persons that they knew? What is done to remember persons who have died and to give emotional support to the living?

Meaning in resident's actions: How would others know if Steve misses Mildred or understands what has happened to her? What are his needs for emotional support?

The role dementia plays: In advance of end-of-life situations, what emotional supports do family members need as they experience changes in the person with dementia that accompany the progression of his/her disease? How do residents' disease progression and deaths affect nursing home staff?

Related sources: Ersek, Kraybill, & Hansberry (2000). Assessing the educational needs and concerns of nursing-home-staff regarding end-of-life care; Wilson & Daly (1999). Family perspectives on dying in long-term care settings; Zilberfein (1999). Coping with death: anticipatory grief and bereavement

What are pros and cons of the following *possible actions?* Are there *other recommendations?*

Possible Actions:

1. Assume that the family's efforts to inform Steve about Mildred's death are sufficient. No further action is needed.
2. Ask the family if they would like staff to further intervene, and follow their advice on this matter. Ask about funeral arrangements and if Steve will be expected to attend.
3. Have one or two staff members who relate best to Steve sit quietly with him and offer sympathy in clear and simple words that recognize this sad event in his life and offer reassurance of continued staff support.
4. Provide opportunities for staff to spend time with Steve—sitting, walking, or in daily activities. Acknowledge that people grieve at the loss of a loved one and talk about what is known of good times the couple shared or positive memories that staff have about Mildred.
5. Inform and give other residents and staff an opportunity to acknowledge Mildred's death. A memorial service may be held.

Commentary on Breaking Bad News

Ethical Considerations

Ethical principles of truth-telling/honesty (veracity) and doing good (beneficence) are at issue. Life is full of situations that involve weighing

the value of truth-telling/acknowledgment of sad or emotionally difficult happenings against whatever pain that may cause. Saying nothing
by way of acknowledgment also may be perceived as uncaring. In this
case, doing good involves meeting the differing needs of many people.

Competing Goods Might Be:

It is good not to withhold information vs. it is good to spare others
    from emotional pain.

It is good to support the wishes of families vs. it is good to know whose
    wishes should prevail when family opinions are divided.

It is good to support the wishes of families vs. it is good to support the
    needs of residents.

Questions

We do not know Steve's feelings related to Mildred's absence or his
sense of what has happened. Does he understand what he has been
told? How can others know? How is he responding? We also may assume,
but do not have an understanding of, how staff and family members
are affected by the loss of Mildred. What feelings have been expressed?

Discussion of *pros and cons of "possible actions"* might be as follows:

Possible Action #1

Assume that the family's efforts to inform Steve about Mildred's death
are sufficient. No further action is needed.

PRO: This action honors values related to family unity and solidarity.
The assumption is that the sadness of the occasion warrants protection
of those involved from the intrusion of others. That is, it may be viewed
as a private family matter.

CON: Because of the couple's history and involvement with others at
New Life Nursing Home, Mildred's death is not a wholly private family
matter. Staff must be concerned about responses of Steve, other residents, and themselves to her loss.

Possible Action #2

Ask the family if they would like staff to further intervene, and follow
their advice on this matter. Ask about funeral arrangements and if Steve
will be expected to attend.

PRO: Staff need to be informed about family wishes and plans so that they can provide support.
CON: The lack of family consensus on how to handle the matter with Steve suggests that they may need more support and time to deal with their own feelings.

Possible Action #3

Have one or two staff members who relate best to Steve sit quietly with him and offer sympathy in clear and simple words that recognize this sad event in his life and offer reassurance of continued staff support.

PRO: This is a respectful, considerate, and compassionate response. It should not be assumed that because others do not know if Steve comprehends the situation, that he has no emotional needs. The use of clear and simple words to communicate with him about his loss also is an expression of honesty and truthfulness about what has taken place and how others feel.
CON: It is possible that Steve could be upset by these communications.

Possible Action #4

Provide opportunities for staff to spend time with Steve—sitting, walking, or in daily activities. Acknowledge that people grieve at the loss of a loved one and talk about what is known of good times the couple shared or positive memories that staff have about Mildred.

PRO: This action assumes that Steve might miss or grieve for Mildred, whether or not his behavior indicates that he does. Spending time offers him caring support and the gift of human companionship. Passage of time together with sustained caring relationships will be better indicators of Steve's special needs for comfort or support.
CON: It is possible that Steve could experience frustration with over-stimulation or change.

Possible Action #5

Inform and give other residents and staff an opportunity to acknowledge Mildred's death. A memorial service may be held.

PRO: This action assumes that other residents and staff may miss or grieve for Mildred. A memorial service is a way to acknowledge and address their needs through the support of a community ritual.

CASE EXAMPLE 3. I'M SCARED OF HIM

Evelyn Clark is a lively 95-year-old woman who was admitted to Azalia Gardens Nursing Home several years ago following a fall at her home that resulted in a fractured hip. Though well recovered, she is largely wheelchair-bound. She has been medically stable throughout her stay, despite chronic conditions that include hypertension, heart disease, and degenerative arthritis. She also is hard of hearing and, alternately, adjusts her hearing aid or removes it altogether while cupping one hand to her ear and loudly repeating, "What? What did you say? I didn't hear what you said. I can't hear, you know." Miss Clark never married and regularly reminds staff that she is "all alone in the world." Consequently, some make an effort to spend extra time with her, since she has no immediate family and few visitors. She is "Evelyn" to all, and she likes to entertain others in her room with her large postcard collection. Many cards were collected on her extensive travels. Each has a story.

Evelyn is very alert and mobile, keeping up with all the latest gossip. She favors interactions with staff and, generally, is agreeable with other residents, unless they happen to be a current roommate. A succession of roommates has come and gone, discouraged by Evelyn's complaints, criticisms, and encroachment on their space.

Lately, Evelyn has been pulling staff aside to voice her concerns about another resident, Mr. Nichols. Mr. Nichols was admitted more recently with a diagnosis of Alzheimer's disease. Though walking unsteadily with a walker at first, he soon was confined to a wheelchair with a rollbar restraint to limit wandering and the potential of falls. He is able to move the chair with his feet and spends much of his time in the dining room or in the hallway near the nurses' station. He seldom verbalizes and does not interact much with others. But Evelyn insists that he has threatened her many times. "He says, 'I'm gonna get you,' and he shakes his fist at me," she reports. "I'm scared of him."

Some staff members sympathize with Evelyn. Even though there are no witnesses to the threats that she describes, they are convinced of her sincerity and believe that her fear and apprehension are genuine. In their view, Evelyn's agitated state and her continued talk about finding a weapon to use against Mr. Nichols "if he comes after me again" can only mean that he is antagonizing her in some way.

Other staff members sympathize with Mr. Nichols. They point to Evelyn's history of roommate difficulties as evidence of her lack of tolerance and suggest that this is yet another example of her well-known tendencies to "pick on people" for no apparent reason. They believe that Evelyn may be provoking Mr. Nichols and misleading staff by claiming that his frustrated reactions are self-initiated.

Since staff members are divided in their opinions about who is the innocent victim in this drama, they also are divided in their opinions about what to do about it. Both residents are being observed for signs of trouble, and the word is out to keep the two apart.

POSITIVE RIGHT: DEFINING COMMUNITY NORMS AND VALUES

The immediate issue is the right of both Evelyn and Mr. Nichols to comfortably access shared public space. Preserving individual integrity in terms of personal feelings of security, dignity, and freedom to do as one wishes also is involved. Organizational-level issues include assessing individual requirements for personal space and privacy as well as the overall residential options within the facility for persons who have different environmentally related needs.

Dialogue

Where is the *ethical conflict* or dilemma of *competing goods*?

Are there *questions* brought to mind but not answered by the narrative?

Institutional policies: What are residential unit/room allocation policies and practices?

Meaning in resident's actions: Why might cognitively intact residents be afraid of residents with dementia? What situations might cause residents with dementia to be aggressive toward others? How may a facility's environment influence residents' moods and interactions?

The role dementia plays: What responsibilities do cognitively intact residents have toward residents with dementia? What may be reasons for moving residents with dementia to special care units, away from cognitively intact residents versus reasons to keep them together?

Related sources: R. A. Kane & Caplan (1990). Chap. 5—Good citizen, bad citizen; Barba et al. (2002). Promoting thriving in nursing homes: The Eden Alternative.

What are pros and cons of the following *possible actions*? Are there *other recommendations*?
Possible Actions

1. Someone needs to get to the bottom of this. A system of surveillance should be established so that there can be an objective

point of view about what is going on and who is instigating the reported confrontations.

2. Evelyn, as the more competent of the two residents, needs to understand that she cannot hold Mr. Nichols responsible for his actions. Her mistreatment of and impatience with roommates in the past raises further doubts about the correctness of her account. A person in authority needs to talk with Evelyn about the importance of being tolerant toward other less competent residents.

3. The behavior of people with dementia often is upsetting to more competent residents. Mr. Nichols should be evaluated for possible transfer to another floor.

4. The cause of Evelyn's distress is not fully clear. She should be encouraged to talk in more detail about what is troubling her and what she thinks ought to be done about it.

5. There is not enough information about the nature of Mr. Nichols's behavior as it relates to Evelyn. He needs to be approached about her concerns, and his responses and reactions should be taken into consideration.

Commentary on I'm Scared of Him

Ethical Considerations

Ethical principles of respect for personal freedom (autonomy) and fairness (justice) are at issue, that is, respect for Evelyn's autonomy and fairness to Mr. Nichols. A background issue in this case also concerns fairness for cognitively intact residents who live on the same residential unit as those who are cognitively impaired. What are the limits of tolerance in such a situation?

Competing Goods Might Be:

It is good to respect Evelyn's need to have some control over her environment.

It is good to respect Mr. Nichols's right to be in the same environment as Evelyn.

Questions

What are Evelyn's and Mr. Nichols's daily routines? What do they enjoy? How might either one or both be redirected to focus attention on other persons and activities?

Does the nursing home environment provide adequate space, stimulating activities, and the kinds of comfortable aesthetic features that may counteract resident confrontations stemming from such things as loneliness, helplessness, and boredom?

Are residents able to distance themselves from individuals who get on their nerves?

Discussion of *pros and cons of "possible actions"* might be as follows:

Possible Action #1

Someone needs to get to the bottom of this. A system of surveillance should be established so that there can be an objective point of view about what is going on and who is instigating the reported confrontations.

PRO: Since no one, other than Evelyn, has reported witnessing a confrontation, observation of both residents seems reasonable.
CON: The fact that staff members already have taken sides on this issue raises doubts as to how "objective" they might be able to be, and what a "system of surveillance" would entail is not clear. Might it be considered invasion of privacy? What will it accomplish to know who is the culprit? What would be done if it was known?

Possible Action #2

Evelyn, as the more competent of the two residents, needs to understand that she cannot hold Mr. Nichols responsible for his actions. Her mistreatment of and impatience with roommates in the past raises further doubts about the correctness of her account. A person in authority needs to talk with Evelyn about the importance of being tolerant toward other less competent residents.

PRO: An appeal to Evelyn's better nature might yield surprising results. There is nothing to indicate that this situation is the same as her past experiences with roommates. Her history of intolerance toward others seems to have involved use of private, not public, space.
CON: Evelyn's history of impatience with others should not be the basis for judging her truthfulness about this issue. Additionally, an authoritarian approach to end the matter is unlikely to work, seems heavy-handed, and is premature, since little is known about what is going on.

Possible Action #3

The behavior of people with dementia often is upsetting to more competent residents. Mr. Nichols should be evaluated for possible transfer to another floor.

PRO: Ongoing evaluation to determine best locations for residents is appropriate.
CON: On the basis of the information that we have, entertaining the notion of possible transfer of Mr. Nichols to another floor seems premature.

Possible Action #4

The cause of Evelyn's distress is not fully clear. She should be encouraged to talk in more detail about what is troubling her and what she thinks ought to be done about it.

PRO: Taking Evelyn's concerns seriously shows respect for her as a person. Understanding what it is about Mr. Nichols that troubles her might help to explain her strong reactions. Talking with someone Evelyn knows and trusts could help her to evaluate her feelings and reactions.
CON: Evelyn may not want to say, or may not have insight into, what is troubling her.

Possible Action #5

There is not enough information about the nature of Mr. Nichols's behavior as it relates to Evelyn. He needs to be approached about her concerns, and his responses and reactions should be taken into consideration.

PRO: Approaching Mr. Nichols in an effort to understand his involvement with Evelyn from his point of view is a sign of fairness and respect for him as a person. The difference in communication skills between the two residents should not prevent Mr. Nichols from being included in an investigation of the matter.
CON: Mr. Nichols may be distressed about Evelyn's accusations, or he even may experience feelings of paranoia.

CASE EXAMPLE 4. IT FEELS JUST LIKE JAIL

Marjorie Shaffer is an 87-year-old resident of Mountain View Villa who has a diagnosis of mid-stage Alzheimer's disease. For 18 months her husband took responsibility for her care with around-the-clock assistance of home health aides. Her nursing home admission was prompted by increased bouts of agitation, constant walking, pacing, and wandering. She has been a resident of Mountain View for ten weeks.

Mrs. Shaffer's behavior on the special care unit is similar to that experienced at home. However, she knows that she is not at home and she strides vigorously from exit to exit, setting off alarms in her wake. She lingers at the elevators and attempts to slip aboard. However, when her husband comes to visit, he is able to distract her from her focus on escape, and they stroll arm-in-arm around and around the floor, talking and laughing softly together. Staff members never know whether they will get a happy nod, a slap on the arm, or a kick in the posterior from Mrs. Shaffer as she passes by. There is neither pattern nor explanation for these gestures. And since Mrs. Shaffer is swift, agile, and strong for her small size, people tend to step aside when they see her coming.

In contrast to her aggressive behavior toward staff, Mrs. Shaffer ignores other residents, with the exception of Grace Horton, whom she constantly follows about. Mrs. Horton's family has complained that Grace finds Marjorie's attentions to be annoying and, occasionally, Mrs. Horton will tell Mrs. Shaffer to "go away." But, generally, Mrs. Shaffer ignores these requests, and Mrs. Horton permits Mrs. Shaffer to accompany her around the floor and follow her into her room, even though the two are not roommates.

One evening Mrs. Horton was found sitting on the floor beside her bed in a pool of urine. Mrs. Shaffer was pulling and tugging on her arms while explaining: "I'm just trying to help my mother into bed." Since that time, staff members have been more vigilant in their efforts to keep the two apart, although the nature of the special care unit makes this very difficult. Recreation staff members have been trying to engage Mrs. Shaffer in planned activities, which she at times will attend, but her attention span is short. Although attempts are made to return her to activities when she wanders away, she often resists and refuses to participate further.

While a social worker was introducing a new resident and his family to the unit one day, Mrs. Shaffer walked up to the group and announced: "You won't like it here. It feels just like jail." Several nursing assistants responded by pointing out some of the attractive features of Mountain View Villa: "Why, Marjorie. Don't you remember the walk we took in the garden yesterday? Didn't you like watching all the birds and smelling the flowers?" . . . "And, you know the food is good here. At least you say so; and you eat everything on your plate and ask for more." . . . "This isn't like jail. This is a nice place. We're all friends here" . . . "Why are you saying it feels just like jail? Don't say that!" [Mrs. Shaffer is hugged and kissed as she is led away.] "You know better. We love you. You know that, don't you?" Mrs. Shaffer allows herself to be removed by the trio of nursing assistants, reaching out to deliver a resounding smack to the seat of the pants of the medication nurse as they walk by. She smiles at the nurse's response ["Ouch, Marjorie. That hurt."], but she says nothing.

NEGATIVE RIGHT: TEMPERING THE CULTURE OF SURVEILLANCE AND RESTRAINT

The issue is one of individual rights not to be restrained, confined, or intruded upon. Creating a comfortable, enjoyable human environment is the organizational-level issue.

Dialogue

Where is the *ethical conflict* or dilemma of *competing goods*?

Are there *questions* brought to mind but not answered by the narrative?

Institutional policies: What are policies and practices related to care of residents with dementia who wander and attempt to escape?

Meaning in resident's actions: What factors may be exacerbating Mrs. Shaffer's wandering, agitation, and aggressive behavior? Why may she have an attachment to Mrs. Horton? What may be encouraging her efforts to escape? How may an unlocked door or free access to a secure area reduce the risk of elopement for residents with dementia?

The role dementia plays: Why can social and environmental changes make wandering worse? What interventions provide positive sensory stimulation, socialization, and exercise to decrease boredom, loneliness, and disorientation? What environmental treatments promote relaxation and improved socialization?

Related sources: Chitsey, Haight, & Jones (2002). Snoezelen: A multisensory environmental intervention; Detweiler, Trinkle, & Anderson (2002). Wander gardens: Expanding the dementia treatment environment; Peatfield, Futrell, & Cox (2002). Wandering: An integrative review; Vollen (1996). Coping with difficult resident behaviors takes time.

What are pros and cons of the following *possible actions*? Are there *other recommendations*?

Possible Actions:

1. Mrs. Shaffer is exhibiting problematic behavior that is not uncom-
    mon in persons at her level of dementia. It might be in her best
    interests to prescribe medication to decrease her agitation and
    elevate her mood.
2. Mrs. Shaffer obviously is depressed, and it might be a good idea
    to obtain a psychiatric evaluation.
3. Mrs. Shaffer needs a friend whom she can trust. It might help
    to identify which staff members she seems to like the most and
    have one of them work at establishing a closer personal relation-
    ship. This could, over time, yield ideas about what approaches
    to care may be most successful and have the best effect.
4. Mrs. Shaffer needs to care for someone or something. She might
    like a cuddly stuffed animal or doll to nurture and have as a
    companion.

Commentary *on* It Feels Just Like Jail

Ethical Considerations

Ethical principles of respect for self-determination (autonomy), preventing harm to others (beneficence), and truthfulness (veracity) are
at issue. It is important to respect Mrs. Shaffer's need for self-determination, but this cannot jeopardize the well-being of other residents. The
question of truth involves the differences between Mrs. Shaffer's opinion
of Mountain View Villa and what others believe (or want her to believe)
to be the truth of the matter.

Competing Goods Might Be:

It is good to allow Mrs. Shaffer freedom to move and express herself.
It is good to protect residents from the unwanted attentions of other
    residents.

It is good to prevent abuse and harm to staff.
It is good to relieve Mrs. Shaffer's distress.

Questions

What should we make of the interaction between Mrs. Shaffer and the
three nursing assistants? What might be alternative ways to respond
to her?

Assuming that the nursing home takes pride in providing excellent care and service in a loving and comfortable environment, can we discount Mrs. Shaffer's perception that it feels just like jail? What is the truth of the matter? Whose truth matters?

Discussion of *pros and cons of "possible actions"* might be as follows:

Possible Action #1

Mrs. Shaffer is exhibiting problematic behavior that is not uncommon in persons at her level of dementia. It might be in her best interests to prescribe medication to decrease her agitation and elevate her mood.

PRO: Some people do need behavior-controlling drugs at a particular stage of their illness. Mrs. Shaffer's physician may want to target specific behaviors where medication might help. If medications are used, atypical antipsychotics are effective for many kinds of behavioral disturbances and have fewer side effects than traditional neuroleptics (e.g., see Tune, 2001).

CON: Older people and people with dementia are very sensitive to medications, and physicians cannot always balance the dose at which a medication will be most effective against unwanted side effects. Finding an effective behavioral approach to address concerns would eliminate the need for medication and the risks that may accompany this type of intervention.

Possible Action #2

Mrs. Shaffer obviously is depressed, and it might be a good idea to obtain a psychiatric evaluation.

PRO: Psychiatric consultation is helpful whenever depression is suspected. Depression can make dementia worse, and, once diagnosed, effective treatments are available.

CON: Psychiatric consultation should not be the automatic response to challenging behavior. What evidence might cause one to conclude that Mrs. Shaffer "obviously is depressed"?

Possible Action #3

Mrs. Shaffer needs a friend whom she can trust. It might help to identify which staff members she seems to like the most and have one of them work at establishing a closer personal relationship. This could, over time, yield ideas about what approaches to care may be most successful and have the best effect.

PRO: A positive relationship between Mrs. Shaffer and one staff member may help relieve the stress on all. She seems to obtain some satisfaction in strolling with her husband and following Mrs. Horton about. Therefore, rechanneling some of that energy into finding things to do with a friendly staff member may be helpful and provide ideas about what approaches to her care may be the most successful.
CON: This represents a greater time commitment on the part of the staff member and may not be feasible, given available nursing home resources.

Possible Action #4

Mrs. Shaffer needs to care for someone or something. She might like a cuddly stuffed animal or doll to have as a companion.

PRO: The idea is worth considering if Mrs. Shaffer indicates interest and has a choice in the matter. Stuffed animals and dolls have been used successfully to comfort and ease distress of elderly nursing home residents. She might transfer undesired attention toward Mrs. Horton to caring for this object.
CON: Stuffed animals and dolls should not be used in place of human relationships. The idea also may seem demeaning to family and others. Other diversions may be as effective or more appreciated and, thus, more appropriate.

CASE EXAMPLE 5. NIGHT AND DAY

Martin Miller is a 90-year-old man with Alzheimer's disease whose wife brought him to River Bend Nursing Home when she could no longer care for him at home. He has been in residence about three months. Mr. Miller dozes through much of the day and is awake and wandering about in the late night–early morning hours. Prior to his admission, his wife discovered that he was leaving the house and wandering around town. "At first, I didn't realize it," she said, "because he'd find his way back home again. He probably didn't go very far. Then he would tell me about his experience the next day . . . that he got lost and so forth. So I'd try to stay awake, but I couldn't . . . This one night, I got up, though. It was three o'clock in the morning, and no Martin; and I thought, 'Well, he'll find his way back again,' which he didn't. I gave it about a half an hour or almost an hour. I had to call the police to look for him." Mrs. Miller employed aides to stay through the night, but it soon became apparent that they could not manage. "He is a big man," Mrs. Miller explained, "and they just couldn't handle him."

At River Bend, Mr. Miller's nocturnal ramblings continue. He works swiftly in his room, emptying dresser drawers and closets of their contents. After piling everything belonging to himself and his roommate onto his bed, he then begins to wander around the unit collecting additional items from other residents' rooms to add to the heap. Since he is very quiet, staff members are not always aware of this activity until his project is well underway. Although he generally is an agreeable person, he can become belligerent over attempts to distract or redirect him. However, offers of food often are effective.

Mr. and Mrs. Miller's son thinks that the nursing home should do something about his father's day/night reversal. He is concerned that he may be sleeping through mealtime and not getting enough to eat. He and his mother take turns assisting Mr. Miller with his noontime meal. "But there is this concern," he explains, "that if we didn't do it and, basically, force him to eat, would somebody else look at him and say, 'Oh, he's asleep; I'm not going to feed him,' you know? He doesn't communicate [about feelings and needs], so if he sleeps through a meal, he can't tell anybody when he wakes up that he's hungry." The family also would like to see Mr. Miller awake for their visits during the day. Mrs. Miller says, "Many times when I come at noon, he's fast asleep; but nobody tells you if he's been up all night. I know he's unruly and won't sleep at the right times. I'd like to have him regulated so that we can talk to him and he can go to activities during the day. Give him coffee to wake him up. Nothing happens at night. What medicines do you have to keep him from sleeping at the wrong time?"

Staff members have been discussing the fact that there are a number of residents who are active throughout the night shift and sleep during much of the day. Not all of them have a diagnosis of dementia, but many, like Mr. Miller, do. There is disagreement over how to deal with this phenomenon. Some individuals think that putting residents to bed by a certain hour and administering medication to help them sleep is an important thing to do. Others think that residents' diverse sleep-wake cycles should be accepted and that the nursing home needs to accommodate to their needs for nourishment, comfort, and socialization both night and day.

POSITIVE RIGHT: PRESERVING INDIVIDUAL INTEGRITY

The issue is one of Mr. Miller's right to do as he wishes.

Dialogue

Where is the *ethical conflict* or dilemma of *competing goods*?

Are there *questions* brought to mind but not answered by the narrative?

Institutional policies: Does the nursing home have a standard care plan for residents with abnormal sleep-awake patterns? Use of a behavioral flow chart with planned interventions may promote healthy sleep-awake patterns without the use of medication.

Meaning in resident's actions: How may differences between home and nursing home living environments account for resident sleep-wake cycle disturbances? How may lifelong habits, age, depression, anxiety, drugs, and medical conditions affect residents' sleep-wake cycles?

The role dementia plays: What interventions may help to increase nocturnal sleep for residents with dementia? What interventions may help to decrease daytime sleepiness?

Related sources: McCrae & Lichstein (2002). Managing insomnia in long-term care; Richards, Sullivan, Phillips, Beck, & Overton-McCoy (2001). The effect of individualized activities on the sleep of nursing home residents who are cognitively impaired; O'Rourke, Klaasen, & Sloan (2001). Redesigning nighttime care for personal care residents; Schnelle, Alessi, Al-Samarrai, Fricker, & Ouslander (1999). The nursing home at night: Effects of an intervention on noise, light, and sleep.

What are pros and cons of the following *possible actions?* Are there *other recommendations?*

Possible Actions:

1. Volunteer to help Mr. Miller unpack the drawers and closets. While joining in, ask questions that may provide clues about what this activity means to him.
2. Arrange to have snacks/mini-meals for residents available to the night shift staff. Before Mr. Miller begins to raid other residents' rooms, ask if he would like to take a break, and offer food.
3. Ask Mr. Miller's physician to prescribe medication to promote sleep.
4. Ask Mr. Miller's family about his past work, hobbies, and interests. Formulate and test ideas for an alternate nighttime activity that might appeal to Mr. Miller because of its close association with his past activities.
5. Discuss pros and cons of trying to change Mr. Miller's sleep-awake cycles with his family.
6. Communicate with Mr. Miller's family about how his nutritional needs are being met.

Commentary on Night and Day

Ethical Considerations

Ethical principles of respecting freedom of choice (autonomy) and providing beneficial care (beneficence) are at issue. It is a question of determining whether it is better to plan care around Mr. Miller's self-determined patterns or to intervene to try to create a more healthful pattern.

Competing Goods Might Be:

It is good to respect Mr. Miller's choice to sleep and to be up and about as he chooses.
It is good to encourage healthful sleep-awake patterns.

Questions

When are residents put to bed for the night? Do staff workloads determine this? For example, a nursing assistant with 7–8 residents who goes off duty at 9:30 p.m., or one who must make rounds at 10 p.m. before going off duty, may start putting residents to bed at early as 7 p.m. Residents who go to sleep at 7 p.m. and are awake at 2 a.m., have had enough sleep. But, if they stay awake through the early morning hours, they will be sleepy later in the day.

What can be done during the day and into the evening to promote sleep at night, for example, encouraging recreational activity and socialization; limiting daytime naps (e.g. no more than two for 30 minutes each); keeping the resident awake as much as possible until after 9 p.m.?

Discussion of *pros and cons of "possible actions"* might be as follows:

Possible Action #1

Volunteer to help Mr. Miller unpack the drawers and closets. While joining in, ask questions that may provide clues about what this activity means to him.

PRO: Some people with dementia rummage through drawers and closets. They could be looking for something to do or they may say they are looking for something in particular, packing to go on a trip, or sorting things. Mr. Miller's reason for rummaging might be shared with a helpful volunteer and the potential comfort of positive human contact should not be underestimated.
CON: Rummaging that becomes an end in itself is unlikely to cease just because the logic of the moment is revealed. Diversion from the activity might work, such as suggesting a "more interesting" thing that Mr. Miller could try or a "more important" thing he could do to help someone else. That entails having an alternate activity that would appeal to him. But logic alone will not be successful and interference in what he has chosen to do may not be welcome. Mr. Miller has resisted

redirection in the past. Locking some drawers and closets and leaving others where he may rummage to his heart's content may be a better compromise.

Possible Action #2

Arrange to have snacks/mini-meals for residents available to the night shift staff. Before Mr. Miller begins to raid other residents' rooms, ask if he would like to take a break, and offer food.

PRO: Mr. Miller may be hungry. A light snack followed by an intervention designed to help him sleep may enable him to have a good night's rest. The intervention should include taking him to the bathroom for toileting; taking him to his bed; assisting him in lying down and ensuring his comfort; and staying with him for a few minutes, holding his hand, giving a gentle back rub, and speaking in soothing tones that encourage sleep. He may have confused night and day and may need to be reminded that it is night.
CON: Too much food, as well as certain foods and beverages, may encourage Mr. Miller's wakefulness instead of putting him in a better mode for sleep. The dietician can suggest appropriate portions and choices of refreshment.

Possible Action #3

Ask Mr. Miller's physician to prescribe medication to promote sleep.

PRO: An effective medication may be found or adjustment of current medication may help. For instance, if Mr. Miller is taking a tranquilizing drug to control his behavior, discussing the possibility of giving the major dose in the evening instead of spreading it out across the day might facilitate sleep with still enough behavior control during the day.
CON: Individuals respond differently to medication, and finding the right type and amount of sedation can be tricky. Older people are more susceptible to side effects than younger people, and sedation makes some people more confused, more sleepy during the day, and, consequently, more likely to fall. It is important to try to find other ways to help a person sleep.

Possible Action #4

Ask Mr. Miller's family about his past work, hobbies, and interests. Formulate and test ideas for an alternate nighttime activity that might appeal to Mr. Miller because of its close association with his past activities.

PRO: It may be possible to replicate some of Mr. Miller's usual routines by identifying elements of work or pastimes that could fit his current patterns. For example, he may need a project or a familiar ritual, like watching the late show, before going to bed. Some people have been in the habit of falling asleep while listening to all-night radio programs. It is worthwhile to find out what Mr. Miller's long-established patterns were.

CON: Returning to past routines may no longer benefit Mr. Miller at this stage of his disease.

Possible Action #5

Discuss pros and cons of trying to change Mr. Miller's sleep-awake cycles with his family.

PRO: A social approach to the issue emphasizes resident autonomy and the importance of having nighttime alternatives to whatever may be missed during daytime napping. Other approaches emphasize changing patterns of day-night reversal through the use of medications or behavioral interventions, as discussed above. The key to what should be done rests with the individual resident. Best answers must be found on a case-by-case basis. That is why collaboration with concerned family members is so important. There needs to be agreement that the best approach for a particular resident is one that will serve his/her best interests.

CON: The difficulties with this approach, if done honestly and well, are that what is found to work best for a particular resident may be counter to family wishes (if the person is a true night owl) or inconvenient for the staff (if a rigorous behavioral approach to prevent serious consequences of sleep deprivation seems in order). The consequences of sleep deprivation are increased risk of falls, increased agitation, weight loss, and muscle aches and pain from the stress of being up and the lack of adequate rest.

Possible Action #6

Communicate with Mr. Miller's family about how his nutritional needs are being met.

PRO: Family concerns about meeting nutritional needs are valid. If Mr. Miller is sleeping through meals or is not eating adequately as a result of fatigue, something will need to be done. Information about established ways of monitoring nutritional status and the results of Mr. Miller's evaluations need to be shared with the family. It will be important to determine if nutritional problems are linked with the sleep-awake pattern issue or constitute a separate issue.

CASE EXAMPLE 6. AS I REMEMBER HIM

Eugene Kaplan is an 84-year-old man who has been living at Clover Hill Estate for two years. His daughter admitted him to this long-term-care facility after his wife's death because her father's progressive dementia limited his ability to live alone and care for himself. She describes her father as a meticulous person who always was very concerned about his appearance. "He could never let anyone see him unshaven," she reports. "Sometimes he would shave twice. He was always looking at himself in the mirror, asking things like, 'Do I look all right? Do you think I need a haircut?' And he was very particular about his clothing. I can remember him asking, in the morning before leaving for work, 'Should I wear this tie, or this tie?' And Mom would say, 'I think this goes best with your outfit.' And he'd say, 'You really think so?' and then they'd argue about it for ten minutes. Because, you see, it had to be just right. He had to have a certain look. He was very, very fussy about how he appeared in public, and concerned about what others would think of him. Even at home, he was not one to sit around and not look nice. Even when he was doing yard work, the minute he came in he had to clean up and get out of dirty clothes."

Mr. Kaplan is able to feed himself, but sometimes he misses his mouth, and food falls on his clothing or on the floor. He also is incontinent of urine, and, despite best efforts, his clothes become wet and need to be changed. His daughter understands these things, but, nevertheless, finds it distressing to visit and find him not clean. "I know he can't be clean every minute of the day," she says. "But I want to see him as I remember him."

Personal hygiene also is an issue. "Being well-shaven," she says, "and good oral hygiene, and his nasal hair trimmed . . . I think there's no excuse for not doing that. And, I think being sure that those things are taken care of is a way of showing respect for him as a person . . . knowing that if he were able to do it for himself, this is the way he would want it done. If he were more aware, he would be so ashamed and appalled to know that he looks the way he does sometimes when I come in to see him."

Mr. Kaplan's daughter takes care of his laundry and color-coordinates his clothing "so that everything matches." She puts outfits together that she thinks are in accord with her father's standards of dress and requests that these choices she makes on his behalf be honored. Often they are; sometimes they are not. The nursing assistants that care for Mr. Kaplan have different views about the relative importance of following the dress code established by Mr. Kaplan's daughter. Some point out that organization of the clothing falls apart when they have to grab something quickly because Mr. Kaplan has had an accident and "needs to be changed fast so that he looks nice for his daughter." Some believe that they care every bit as much as Mr. Kaplan's daughter about the way he looks and that they are able to put together outfits that look good on him without any help from her. Others think that, although these attempts to organize their work do not allow them to dress Mr. Kaplan as they wish, it is not that difficult to humor her in order to maintain peace. Thus, the daughter's satisfaction with Mr. Kaplan's appearance varies daily with the philosophy of whichever nursing assistant has been assigned to care for him.

POSITIVE RIGHT: PRESERVING INDIVIDUAL INTEGRITY

The issue is one of respect for Mr. Kaplan's dignity and basic human needs. Care and respect for the resident's family also needs to be considered.

Dialogue

Where is the *ethical conflict* or dilemma of *competing goods?*

Are there *questions* brought to mind but not answered by the narrative?

Institutional policies: What are the policies and standards related to cleanliness, grooming, and appropriate manner of dress for residents?

Meaning in resident's actions: What do issues with eating and continence suggest in terms of present and future care needs?

The role dementia plays: What is evidence of self-neglect as a result of disease and disability versus willful or unintentional neglect on the part of other persons? What is the daughter's appropriate role in Mr. Kaplan's care?

Related sources: Janzen (2001). Long-term care for older adults: The role of the family; Kelly, Swanson, Maas, & Tripp-Reimer (1999). Family visitation on special care units; Curry, Porter, Michalski, & Gruman

(2000). Individualized care: perceptions of certified nursing assistants.

What are pros and cons of the following *possible actions?* Are there *other recommendations?*

Possible Actions:

1. Talk with Mr. Kaplan's daughter about how dementia changes people. Remind her that Mr. Kaplan is not the same as she remembers him and that what used to be important to him may not be so important to him now.
2. Investigate routines around shaving and personal hygiene to learn more about what helps or hinders this part of Mr. Kaplan's care.
3. Ask Mr. Kaplan's daughter for extra clothing that nursing assistants can use to "mix-and-match" with what Mr. Kaplan is wearing when a quick change is needed.
4. Ask Mr. Kaplan's daughter if she has photographs of her father in a variety of situations that can be displayed in his room to orient staff members to his life before Clover Hill.
5. Involve Mr. Kaplan's regularly assigned nursing assistant(s) and Mr. Kaplan's daughter in discussion about his perceived needs related to dressing activities.

Commentary on As I Remember Him

Ethical Considerations

Ethical principles of faithfulness/loyalty (fidelity) and respectful care (beneficence) are at issue. Mr. Kaplan's daughter is being loyal to her father by attending to remembered preferences and personal values that he can no longer express and enforce for himself. She asks that staff comply out of respect for him. However, what constitutes respectful care becomes an issue when family and care providers' daily care priorities differ.

Potential and actual neglect of residents always must be considered in situations where caregivers are busy and staffing is inadequate. Dealing with family concerns and staff member frustration (or lack of awareness/concern) is another ethical consideration.

Competing Goods Might Be:

It is good to faithfully respect what was important to a resident in his/her past.

It is good to understand and respect families' needs to be loyal to their family member.

It is good to set priorities that are in the current best interests of the resident.

Questions

We do not know the extent to which Mr. Kaplan has been given opportunities to participate in and make choices about his grooming and apparel. It is possible, however, that he has progressed beyond the point where he can do this. If so, how might he still be engaged in the decision-making process?

We know about the daughter's views and the different nursing assistant responses that it elicits. But we do not know much about patterns of interaction. Who talks to whom, and what is the nature of the conversations? What is the relationship between family members and staff? Are families treated as members of the care team? What does such membership mean and entail?

Does Mr. Kaplan need more mealtime assistance (e.g., see Kayser-Jones & Schell, 1997a, 1997b)? Does his problem with incontinence need to be evaluated (e.g., see Jirovec & Wells, 1990; Ouslander, 2000)? See also Kayser-Jones (2000) for an example of the unethical treatment of a resident whose health and dignity were compromised through lack of attention to basic human care needs.

Discussion of *pros and cons of "possible actions"* might be as follows:

Possible Action #1

Talk with Mr. Kaplan's daughter about how dementia changes people. Remind her that Mr. Kaplan is not the same as she remembers him and that what used to be important to him may not be so important to him now.

PRO: It may be appropriate to talk about change if, indeed, Mr. Kaplan's behavior has changed, for example, if he sometimes refuses efforts to help him shave or dress. This may account for why he is not always looking his best.

CON: If refusal of care is not an issue, showing respect for what is known about Mr. Kaplan's past personality and individual preferences by attending to personal hygiene (which should be considered mandatory) and being sure that he is well-dressed according to his daughter's wishes does not seem like too much to ask.

Possible Action #2

Investigate routines around shaving and personal hygiene to learn more about what helps or hinders this part of Mr. Kaplan's care.

PRO: It is important for the care supervisor/team leader to observe or inquire in a nonjudgmental way about needs to help nursing assistants with Mr. Kaplan's routine care. For example, it will help if shaving equipment is available and in good repair.
CON: Care will be hindered if, for example, a nursing assistant is worried about being bitten when providing oral care. Or, is workload an issue? Though nursing assistants are generally encouraged to report problems they may be having in delivering care to residents, they may feel that no one will understand, that they may be criticized, that help is not available, or that there are some situations that are beyond anyone's help. If there is any truth to those possibilities, those are matters that should be taken very seriously.

Possible Action #3

Ask Mr. Kaplan's daughter for extra clothing that nursing assistants can use to "mix-and-match" with what Mr. Kaplan is wearing when a quick change is needed.

PRO: Flexibility in the dress code that allows nursing assistants some choices, too, when it really matters could help to ease the situation.
CON: This suggestion may be perceived as challenging a valued role in Mr. Kaplan's care that is very important to the daughter.

Possible Action #4

Ask Mr. Kaplan's daughter if she has photographs of her father in a variety of situations that can be displayed in his room to orient staff members to his life before Clover Hills.

PRO: Staff members are likely to genuinely appreciate glimpses of residents' earlier lives. Photographs can capture some personal qualities, obscured by illness, to which family members desire to be faithful. This action may help staff members come to know Mr. Kaplan in a new way and to understand and appreciate his daughter's point of view.

Possible Action #5

Involve Mr. Kaplan's regularly assigned nursing assistant(s) and Mr. Kaplan's daughter in discussion about his perceived needs related to dressing activities.

PRO: When a nursing home admits a resident, the responsibility to care for family members is an implicit part of the transition. Family members entrust the resident to the nursing home's care, expecting to remain involved, but families also have needs of their own. In Mr. Kaplan's case, the need to respect his personal lifetime values and to support his daughter's faithfulness to her memories of them are strongly intertwined. Enlisting staff support for Mr. Kaplan's daughter around preserving her father's dignity, in accordance with her remembrances, is an act of kindness and compassion that takes both them and the enormity of their situation into account.

CON: It is possible that the daughter is over-involved, controlling, and/or unrealistic, and she may need help with the transition from primary protector and caregiver to more of a shared role with nursing home staff.

CASE EXAMPLE 7. TIMING IS EVERYTHING

Irma Gillis is an 81-year-old woman who came to Mayville Manor a year ago when her worsening dementia had taken its toll on her daughters, one of whom had moved into her house to care for her. "I couldn't do it," this daughter explained. "You know, as the disease progresses, you start not being able to do as much. You can't bribe them; you can't coax them. Nothing means anything. When I would give her a bath, I'd have to get in the tub with her, and she'd say 'No! No way!' And she'd be all soap, and I wouldn't know what I was going to do. I found myself shouting at her . . . for what? . . . because I wanted to help her. She couldn't stay soapy. I was just gonna take a minute. I'd be done soon. 'No way! No! No!' And there was nothing I could say. I just couldn't reason with her. I was fighting stuff all the time 'cause there's no rhyme or reason to anything she does."

At Mayville, Irma awakes at dawn and by 6 a.m. or earlier, is sitting in the dining room, wearing socks and a nightgown and asking for coffee. A night shift staff member brings her a cup, and the day shift finds her cheerfully sipping and looking out the window. The cheerful mood disappears, however, at the suggestion that she return to her room to wash and dress for the day. She insists that she is dressed and even rejects a robe and slippers on the chilliest days. Different staff members try leaving her alone for awhile and coming back to try again, but once she is out of her room, the chances of getting her back without a struggle are slim.

Usually, Mrs. Gillis is left at the dining room table until breakfast is over and several nursing assistants can combine efforts to complete morning care before lunch. They report: "Our biggest fights are over hair. We can't get it washed without a fight; and it does not look good. She gives the hairdresser a hard time too. She can't cut or set it. We put her hair up in rollers and let her go one day; and a few minutes later the rollers were in the toilet. Bathing's always been an issue . . . her toenails getting cut . . . any grooming. She'll hit. And she's got a terrific grip. When she doesn't want something done and she gets her hands on you, she can hurt you."

Mrs. Gillis tells her daughters that people are beating her up. They say that they understand how difficult it is. The one who had cared for her mother at home said, "You can only try so long to get somebody dressed, and when they're mad, you might as well give it up for awhile." The other daughter believes that their mother's anger is justified because of indignities suffered. She said, "I'll never forget the first time the aides took her to the bathroom . . . the fight she put up. She was mad and crying. They were putting diapers on her. I think that she knew what was going on and wasn't having any part of it. It's a terrible indignity and embarrassment to have to go through something like that. I'd cry and be mad too."

Staff members who care for Mrs. Gillis have observed that she does not consistently resist care. She has a particularly warm relationship with a nurse on the evening shift who, according to the staff, "can get her to do almost anything." "Oh, I just love her up, and chat with her awhile and that paves the way," that nurse reports. "But," she adds, "that doesn't mean she'll go along with everything I'd like her to do. It has to be the right person at the right time. Timing is everything." The care team has suggested that the timing of some care routines for Mrs. Gillis, such as bathing and dressing, be moved to other shifts. The goal would be to find a time when she might be more receptive to assistance with her personal care. However, administration has concerns about the ability of more lightly staffed shifts to assume work responsibilities that generally are taken on during the day shifts when staff resources are greater.

NEGATIVE RIGHT: LEARNING THE LIMITS OF INTERVENTION

The issue is one of Mrs. Gillis's right not to be forced to do things.

Dialogue

Where is the *ethical conflict* or dilemma of *competing goods*?

Are there *questions* brought to mind but not answered by the narrative?

Institutional policies: What are standard routines for providing personal care to residents on different shifts? Are there times of the day when residents cannot be bathed, get a meal, or have a snack if they want to? What would an individualized routine for a resident be like? Are there examples where this has been done for others? What were the results?

Meaning in resident's actions: How can former lifestyles influence residents' preferred daily patterns? What environmental factors or care-giver behaviors could be related to Mrs. Gillis's refusal of personal care? What are the objections and alternatives to routine use of "diapers" in the care of nursing home residents?

The role dementia plays: Is refusal of morning care a result of forgetting that it still needs to be completed? Is Mrs. Gillis able to understand requests or instructions associated with care activities? Does she realize that she needs help with her care? What options may be effective in maximizing resident comfort with and acceptance of bathing, dressing, and other personal care activities? Is undiagnosed/untreated pain an issue in care?

Related sources: Hoeffer, Rader, McKenzie, Lavelle, & Stewart (1997). Reducing aggressive behavior during bathing cognitively impaired nursing home residents; Miller (1997). Physically aggressive resident behavior during hygienic care; Kraker & Vajdik (1997). Designing the environment to make bathing pleasant in nursing homes; Curry et al. (2000). Individualized care: perceptions of certified nurse's aides.

What are pros and cons of the following *possible actions?* Are there *other recommendations?*
Possible Actions:

1. Ask the daughters about the routines that Mrs. Gillis has used throughout her life, including usual times of waking up and going to bed, mealtimes, and normal activities.
2. Consider having a member of the night shift staff ready to help Mrs. Gillis wash and dress for the day when she normally awakens and before she leaves her room.
3. Serve the early morning coffee to Mrs. Gillis in her room and let her breakfast there to see if the transition into morning care becomes any easier.
4. Ask the daughters specific questions about past bathing and grooming routines, such as preference for tub or shower, time of day preferred for bathing, familiar rituals around care of hair, such as brushing and home styling vs. patronage of a beauty

salon, curling, permanents, favorite beauty products, and so forth.

5. Explore alternative bathing protocols for a gentler more soothing approach.

6. Explore alternatives in incontinence products to see if an effective alternative to the use of diapers is available.

Commentary on Timing Is Everything

Ethical Considerations

Ethical principles of respect for self-determination (autonomy), doing good (beneficence), and equitable use of resources (justice) are at issue. There is tension between respect for Mrs. Gillis's autonomy and care delivery that meets her needs and does not strain institutional resources.

Competing Goods Might Be:

It is good to allow Mrs. Gillis to establish her own routine.
It is good to maintain routines that allow the nursing home to be operational.
It is good to incorporate resident wishes into the plan of care.
It is good to follow a plan based on professional judgment of resident care needs.

Questions

There is so much about Mrs. Gillis as a person that this short vignette cannot convey. What is her personal history? What sort of woman was she before developing dementia? How could knowing her as she was before help us understand her better now? What are other obstacles to providing individualized care?

Discussion of *pros and cons of "possible actions"* might be as follows:

Possible Action #1

Ask the daughters about the routines that Mrs. Gillis has used throughout her life, including usual times of waking up and going to bed, mealtimes, and normal activities.

PRO: Knowledge of lifetime habits and patterns of activity is important to have as the basis for developing an individualized plan of care.
CON: It may be that Mrs. Gillis has developed some new habits and routines or that these have changed due to the disease process.

Possible Action #2

Consider having a member of the night shift staff ready to help Mrs. Gillis wash and dress for the day when she normally awakens and before she leaves her room.

PRO: This might resolve any early morning tension and provide a calming start to the day.
CON: It may not be feasible.

Possible Action #3

Serve the early morning coffee to Mrs. Gillis in her room and let her breakfast there to see if the transition into morning care becomes any easier.

PRO: Both "Possible Actions" #2 and #3 respect Mrs. Gillis's current preferences. They rest on an assumption that delivery of morning care may be easier if it happens before Mrs. Gillis leaves her room.
CON: Both requests depend on inter-shift communication and consensus on what modifications of nursing home routines may best accommodate her needs. However, concerns that have been raised about the ability of more lightly staffed shifts to take on extra responsibilities make this more than an issue of communication. Staffing may be insufficient at night (a resource issue). Eating breakfast in her room also puts Mrs. Gillis at risk of being left alone and deprives her of the more stimulating environment of the dining room.

Possible Action #4

Ask the daughters specific questions about past bathing and grooming routines, such as preference for tub or shower, time of day preferred for bathing, familiar rituals around care of hair, such as brushing and home styling versus patronage of a beauty salon, curling, permanents, favorite beauty products, and so forth.

PRO: Specific details that go beyond the generalities of habitual practices and lifetime activity patterns are needed to determine just how

much of the nursing home environment and routines will seem foreign and, possibly, threatening to Mrs. Gillis. When timing is everything, one wants to try approaches that may appear most familiar in detail to the person involved.
CON: This approach may not apply or be feasible.

Possible Action #5

Explore alternative bathing protocols for a gentler more soothing approach.

Possible Action #6

Explore available incontinence products for an effective alternative to diapers.

PRO: Both of these actions (Possible Actions #5 and #6) take into consideration the variety of approaches to personal hygiene needs that are available today. These include cleansing agents that require no rinsing and incontinence products that more closely resemble regular underwear.
CON: Cost may be a factor.

CASE EXAMPLE 8. DON'T GET AROUND MUCH ANYMORE

Claude Allen was a world traveler before he was admitted to Rainbow Villa with a diagnosis of Alzheimer's disease. He is a widower and has two sons living in distant states. His only regular visitor is a sister, who is ten years his junior. While in the earlier stages of his disease, Mr. Allen adjusted to nursing home routines and became an active participant in planned events and activities. He especially enjoyed fieldtrips, discussion groups, and music. Two years later, however, the decision was made to move 80-year-old Mr. Allen to the special care unit because of behavior that had become intolerable to fellow residents on the floor to which he originally had been admitted. Mr. Allen had begun to wander into other resident's rooms, take their belongings, and sleep in their beds. Their angry responses produced confusion and embarrassment on Mr. Allen's part. He would try to respond verbally, but his deteriorating language abilities would not allow for clear expression of thought. He became increasingly reclusive and withdrawn.

On the special care unit, Mr. Allen continues to keep to himself, spending most of his time in his room and refusing to come to the dining room to eat. His sister is concerned about the change in his usual outgoing ways. "I don't think I have ever come up here when he isn't in his room," she says. "Now, I know they say they try to take him to things and that he's participating more, but he won't stay; and if I don't go along to see that he doesn't wander off there is no one who can just sit with him."

Mr. Allen's sister is an advocate of unit-based activities. "Can you think what it would be like if you could hire a recreation person for each floor . . . eight hours on each floor?" she asks. When she brings Mr. Allen to sing-alongs in the dining room, she observes that he will tap his foot in time to the music and hum along with the melody from time to time. But she cannot visit more than once or twice a week. In her absence, the recreation therapists make an effort to involve Mr. Allen in activities, but if he wanders away from groups being taken to programs and events, transportation resources are not always sufficient to seek out and retrieve him.

Rainbow Villa's practice is to invite but not to force residents to attend programs and social events. Therefore, staff members are tolerant of Mr. Allen's tendency to decline and walk away from most activities. They reassure his sister that they will continue to encourage his participation as much as possible. This is not enough to calm her fears. "If you don't use it, you lose it," she says. "I think all these people could use more activity. There are some people [residents] who haven't gone downhill at all; and, these are the ones who are mobile and participating. They have to have something going on in their lives. They can't just sit there all day long. The ones who are active are not changing."

POSITIVE RIGHT: DEFINING COMMUNITY NORMS AND VALUES

The issue is one of Mr. Allen's right to attend community events, have opportunities to form relationships, pursue activities that are of personal benefit, and, in these ways, to obtain a fair share of goods, services, and amenities. Organizational-level issues include transportation and personnel resources.

Dialogue

Where is the *ethical conflict* or dilemma of *competing goods*?

Are there *questions* brought to mind but not answered by the narrative?

Institutional policies: What types of group and individual activities are available to residents on a regular basis? Are activities appropriate,

sufficiently varied for a range of interests, and leveled to accommodate residents with different functional and cognitive abilities? What
is the ratio of unit-based to facility-wide activities? What personnel
and volunteer resources are available to accompany residents to activities? Are families involved? How is resident participation evaluated?
Are leisure interest profiles completed and updated for individual
residents? Have environmental innovations (e.g., Edenization) to
increase companionship, spontaneity, interest, and variety in residents' lives been considered? What are they?

Meaning in resident's actions: Is Mr. Allen's social withdrawal related to
awareness of or embarrassment over his cognitive impairment and
others' responses to him? Is he depressed? Or is social withdrawal
related to progression of his disease, indicating a need to adjust
activities and assess the level of stimulation that he needs and is able
to tolerate?

The role dementia plays: Is the special care unit over-stimulating or frightening? Are large groups and noisy dining areas too overwhelming
for Mr. Allen? Is he bored, disoriented, or insecure without the
reassuring presence, explanations, and prompting of a companion?
Is he able to understand what invitations to participate in activities
are about? Is there opportunity for activities that match his interests,
abilities, and attention span?

Related sources: Buettner (1998). A team approach to dynamic programming on the special care unit; Jones & Haight (2002). Environmental
transformations.

What are pros and cons of the following *possible actions*? Are there *other
recommendations*?
Possible Actions:

1. This appears to be a resource issue rather than an ethical issue
    and it is difficult to tell from this account how nursing home
    staff might do anything differently. Staff should continue to re-
    assure Mr. Allen's sister that they are making every effort to
    involve him in activities.
2. Involvement of family members is desirable and beneficial to
    residents. Nursing home personnel should make Mr. Allen's
    sister feel very welcome when she visits so that she will be encour-
    aged by their personal interest and enthused about accompa-
    nying Mr. Allen to programs and events.
3. The Director of Volunteer Services may be able to help in individ-
    ual cases such as this where a resident may benefit from a relation-

ship with a volunteer friendly visitor. The goal would be to increase Mr. Allen's participation in activities and to help him regain confidence in socializing with others on the special care unit.

4. Recreational services could reevaluate Mr. Allen to see if he might benefit from some one-on-one recreational activities.

5. Address the issue of resources for transportation and program assistance. Appoint a task force to look into ways in which the facility might assure that more residents get taken to activities and receive sufficient individual support to capture their attention and help hold their interest once they get there.

Commentary *on* Don't Get Around Much Anymore

Ethical Considerations

Ethical principles of doing good (beneficence) and fairness (justice) are at issue. In this case, what is good for some will be less fair to others (i.e., taking more time and resources to mobilize residents like Mr. Allen vs. transporting a larger number of residents that take less time.)

Competing Goods Might Be:

It is good to transport as many residents as possible to activities (the greater good that favors cognitively intact persons who, comparatively speaking, may be assembled and transported more quickly and efficiently).

It is good to keep people with dementia socially active.

Questions

Contextual questions that could have some bearing on Mr. Allen's decreased participation in community activities might be: How do residents get transported to and from off-unit activities? Who is responsible? How many people are needed, on average, and how long does it take to coordinate this effort? How many people can stay through the activity to monitor, sit with residents, and attend to their needs? Are residents with dementia left out or are they the last persons to be taken to activities because of the extra time and attention they may require? Do staff have residents ready on time to be taken to activities? Do staff accept a simple "yes" or "no" response as indication of a resident's desire to participate in an activity or do they take the time to explain and encourage participation? Are assumptions made about residents who often decline invitations to attend activities that result in eventual failure to invite or include them because staff members anticipate refusal?

Discussion of *pros and cons of "possible actions"* might be as follows:

Possible Action #1

This appears to be a resource issue and it is difficult to tell from the point of view of a single individual how nursing home staff might do anything differently. Staff should continue to reassure Mr. Allen's sister that they are making every effort to involve him in activities.

PRO: Resource issues may not be seen as ethical dilemmas amenable to resolution at the level of individuals. That is, the question may be seen as one that relates to the domain of organizational ethics rather than to practice ethics with its focus on individual cases. Thus, for supporters of this point of view, the larger resource issue affecting Mr. Allen is dismissed as an ethical question that needs to be directed elsewhere (e.g., to administration).
CON: However, the effects of organizational arrangements that affect resource allocation at the individual level cannot so easily be dismissed. For example, Jonsen et al. (1998) caution that even though larger issues involving the allocation of scarce medical resources may fall within another ethical domain (e.g., the ethics of health policy) there is still a question of "whether physicians should make allocation decisions by balancing societal efficiency against the interests of individual patients" (p. 182). Similarly, in the face of limited resources, nursing home staff may feel obliged to balance institutional efficiency against the interests of individual residents. Consequently, any resource issue that compromises a resident's quality of life is a legitimate ethical problem of nursing home care in search of a solution at both individual and organizational levels (which means that administration needs to be involved).

Possible Action #2

Involvement of family members is desirable and beneficial to residents. Nursing home personnel should make Mr. Allen's sister feel very welcome when she visits so that she will be encouraged by their personal interest and enthused about accompanying Mr. Allen to programs and events.

PRO: Mr. Allen and his sister might appreciate the personal interest, despite the ulterior motive.

CON: Mr. Allen's sister cannot visit more than once or twice a week. She seems to care about her brother's welfare. It would not do to instill a sense of guilt if she cannot do more.

Possible Action #3

The Director of Volunteer Services may be able to help in individual cases such as this where a resident may benefit from a relationship with a volunteer friendly visitor. The goal would be to increase Mr. Allen's participation in activities and to help him regain confidence in socializing with others on the special care unit.

Possible Action #4

Recreational therapy services could reevaluate Mr. Allen to see if he might benefit from some one-on-one recreational activities.

PRO: Both of these ideas (Possible Actions #3 and #4) are individualized to be of benefit.
CON: If there is a shortage of volunteers or recreation therapists the facility may be too understaffed to provide one-on-one approaches in the form of social and recreational activities.

Possible Action #5

Address the issue of resources for transportation and program assistance. Appoint a task force to look into ways in which the facility might assure that more residents get taken to activities and receive sufficient individual support to capture their attention and help hold their interest once they get there.

PRO: This action represents a commitment on the part of the nursing home to search for creative solutions and to make changes when needed rather than accept the status quo. It illustrates an ethical stance in relation to resident-focused community values.
CON: It may not produce a solution with specific relevance to Mr. Allen's situation.

CASE EXAMPLE 9. A MOVING EXPERIENCE

Carlo DeAngelo is a 79-year-old man who, for four years, has been a resident on the special care unit at Deerpark Estate long-term care facility. His granddaughter, who is his nearest living relative, declares that he has been there the longest of any resident on that floor. "A lot of things have happened to him," she says. "But the heart attack . . . that was the only major medical problem he's had, except for the dementia taking over more and more. He would wander a lot. He lived with my husband and I before he came here, and I couldn't leave him alone. I'd find him walking down the middle of the street. He'd get angry when you'd try to prevent him from going outside; and he was strong. It really was hard, physically. So this floor was good for that wandering around and stuff."

Staff members are especially fond of Mr. DeAngelo. Once free to wander without being challenged, his cheerful and sociable personality blossomed. He was an enthusiastic participant in activities and developed strong attachments to all of the staff on the unit. When his verbal abilities became increasingly impaired, staff made special efforts to interact with him. And, when he became too weak to walk anymore, they wheeled him all around the facility and took him outside in good weather. Following his heart attack, Mr. DeAngelo was in an especially weakened state, requiring total care and transfers between bed and chair with the assistance of a mechanical lift. Although the affection staff members have for him is strong and long-standing, it is apparent that he no longer needs the special benefits that this unit was designed to provide. The care team believes that he will be able to receive more skilled attention on another unit accustomed to providing higher levels of care. But, when they called Mr. DeAngelo's granddaughter to tell her, she expressed serious concerns. "I don't want him to leave," she said. "I really believe he belongs where he is with people who for him, in his present condition, are family. He's bonded with them. He's lost his past. The last time I was able to communicate with him, he was a kid again in his mind. But he knew all the people on the floor who care for him every day. That's what you're taking away from him. The only memory he has anymore is of these people, and that worries me. I believe a change like this, with complete strangers all of a sudden will bother him. He knows who takes care of him. I think he feels comfortable where he is. When he had the heart attack, he could have died then. I thought, 'Well, this is it.' But he bounced back. I believe he wants to be here, because he could have let go and left this earth then. He's old and he's got terrible dementia; but I think his wanting to stay and the happiness he has found with the people on this floor are connected."

Staff members are distressed by the granddaughter's reaction, in part, because some of them also have been questioning whether or not an exception might be made. "He's been here for four years," they point out. "And this floor has been his home for so long, he's like family." The issues revisited are: (1) the resource issue—there are a limited number of beds on the unit that are always in demand for residents whose behavior warrants special attention; and (2) the care issue—staff on other units are more accustomed to and can more readily accommodate the total care needs of Mr. DeAngelo. It is agreed to proceed with trial visits for Mr. DeAngelo on the proposed new floor. He will be accompanied by his regular nursing assistant and his granddaughter.

POSITIVE RIGHT: DEFINING COMMUNITY NORMS AND VALUES

The issue is one of Mr. DeAngelo's right to opportunities to maintain relationships and retain his previously established share of goods, services, and amenities. At the organizational level, the issue is one of allowing individuals to "age in place."

Dialogue

Where is the *ethical conflict* or dilemma of *competing goods*?

Are there *questions* brought to mind but not answered by the narrative?

Institutional policies: How are residents selected for admission to the Special Care Unit (SCU)? What are the policies on aging in place and the criteria for maintaining residence on the unit? Do staff members on other units have knowledge about dementia and specialized training in dementia care similar to that of SCU staff members? What are staff-to-resident ratios on the SCU and other resident units? What hospice or comfort care options are available as Mr. DeAngleo's condition continues to deteriorate?

Meaning in resident's actions: Is it possible to know, without a trial, if relocation to another unit will be upsetting to Mr. DeAngelo versus neutral or even beneficial?

The role dementia plays: How do residents' care needs change toward the ends of their lives? How does care of residents in their final stage of physical decline become more emotionally and physically demanding on family members and staff? How can staff and family members recognize their own grieving and prepare to support each other as progressive decline and death of the resident become more imminent?

Related sources: Kovach (1998). Nursing home dementia care units: Providing a continuum of care rather than aging in place; Maas, Specht, Weiler, Buckwalter, & Turner (1998). Special care units for people with Alzheimer's disease: Only for the privileged few? Weaverdyck, Wittle, & deLaski-Smith (1998). In-place progression: Lessons learned from the Huron Wood's staff; Wilson, Kovach, & Stearns (1996). Hospice concepts in the care for end-stage dementia; Baer & Hanson (2000). Families' perception of the added value of hospice in the nursing home.

What are pros and cons of the following *possible actions?* Are there *other recommendations?*
Possible Actions:

1. Let Mr. DeAngelo sit with his granddaughter and nursing assistant in a communal area in the new environment and closely observe his reactions and responses as he is introduced to people there. Continue close observation for new or different responses on return to his familiar environment.
2. Invite the nursing assistant who will be regularly assigned to Mr. DeAngelo on the new floor to participate with his current nursing assistant in his care so that they may begin to be comfortable with one another.
3. Have Mr. De Angelo's nursing assistant go with him to the new environment to participate with others there in his care a few times to ease the transition from one floor to the other.
4. The granddaughter's reasons for wanting to have Mr. DeAngelo stay in place with staff who have become like an extended family to him are understandable. Petition for an exception in this case to allow him to stay on the floor where he has been for four years.
5. Listen without judgment to the granddaughter's concerns and, if indeed the transition must be made, actively involve her in planning a move that will be most supportive of both her own and Mr. DeAngelo's needs.

Commentary *on* A Moving Experience

Ethical Considerations

Ethical principles of doing good (beneficence), doing no harm (nonmaleficence), and being fair (justice) are at issue. The recommendation for the move is motivated by a desire to provide a more intensive physical care environment that is consistent with Mr. DeAngelo's changing physical needs. However, the concern of Mr. DeAngelo's granddaughter and some staff members is that this may do more harm than good. The regular demand for special care unit beds raises additional concerns about the fairness of Mr. DeAngelo remaining beyond his time to make the best use of that environment when others might need and benefit from it more.

Competing Goods Might Be:

It is good to allow Mr. DeAngelo to age in place on the unit that has become his home.

It is good to see that residents with changing needs for physical care are well placed.

It is good to see that resources are distributed equitably on the basis of need.

Questions

How has the heart attack affected cognition and social interaction? What best defines quality of life: having psychosocial needs met or having physical needs met? And who, in this case, should decide? Who establishes the policy on resident moves? Should there be exceptions?

Discussion of *pros and cons of "possible actions"* might be as follows:

Possible Action #1

Let Mr. DeAngelo sit with his granddaughter and nursing assistant in a communal area in the new environment and closely observe his reactions and responses as he is introduced to people there. Continue close observation for new or different responses on return to his familiar environment.

PRO: This provides an opportunity for Mr. DeAngelo and his granddaughter to experience and respond to the new environment in a gradual, controlled way.
CON: It is a limited exercise that cannot duplicate the magnitude of the change, if it is to occur.

Possible Action #2

Invite the nursing assistant who will be regularly assigned to Mr. DeAngelo on the new floor to participate with his current nursing assistant in his care so that they may begin to be comfortable with one another.

Possible Action #3

Have Mr. DeAngelo's nursing assistant go with him to the new environment to participate with others there in his care a few times to ease the transition from one floor to the other.

PRO: These actions (Possible Action #2 and #3) provide opportunities for adjustment to a change in care providers.
CON: Arrangements will need to be made to coordinate times for the nursing assistants to work together and to cover the "guest" nursing assistant's assignment while she is with Mr. DeAngelo.This approach doubles the resource requirement.

Possible Action #4

The granddaughter's reasons for wanting to have Mr. DeAngelo stay in place with staff who have become like an extended family to him are understandable. Petition for an exception in this case to allow him to stay on the floor where he has been for four years.

PRO: Making an exception in this case would avoid what some fear would be the emotional harm of such a major change.
CON: There is the question of whether this would be doing Mr. DeAngelo a disservice by not moving him to a floor where his physical care needs could receive more attention. It also may be that someone who could benefit from being on the special care unit is being denied the room.

Possible Action #5

Listen without judgment to the granddaughter's concerns and, if indeed the transition must be made, actively involve her in planning a move that will be most supportive of both her own and Mr. DeAngelo's needs.

PRO: This avoids a contest between the nursing home and the granddaughter and validates her perspective on the proposed move. Involving her in the plan will give her a sense of control that may make the transition easier for her and her grandfather.
CON: Care must be taken not to demand more of the granddaughter than she can give at this stressful time, and to avoid the confusion of

seeming to offer her control of matters that may need to remain at the discretion of the nursing home.

CASE EXAMPLE 10. I'M READY TO GO HOME

Eighty-six-year old Jessie Robinson has been a resident of Meadowvale Estate long-term care facility for six months. From her admission to the present time, she always has been nicely dressed and well groomed. And, despite severe confusion and memory problems, she has maintained many social skills, trying hard to follow conversations and respond appropriately, even though in most instances she cannot. She is oriented only to self and requires constant direction due to a short attention span. She has been ambulating independently with a cane, although her balance is poor and she has fallen on occasion.

Mrs. Robinson has two children and five grandchildren. Her son and daughter-in-law live near Meadowvale. They are very supportive and involved in her care. Her daughter's family lives far away in another state. They have visited once, and sister and brother keep in touch through e-mail and phone calls. The son describes his mother as strong and intelligent. She and her husband were high school teachers. On retirement, they traveled extensively and had an active social life until he underwent treatment for lung cancer and died a year later. That same year, Mrs. Robinson's dementia was diagnosed. She lived independently for another four years during which time she gave up driving on her physician's advice and eventually was unable to manage her finances, due to increased cognitive dysfunction. Her son hired 24-hour home services to monitor and assist her. Six months later, her family suggested she move to a nursing home. She, reportedly, was saddened by but accepting of their advice.

Prior to being diagnosed with dementia and seven years prior to her admission, Mrs. Robinson executed a living will. One year before admission she named her son as her health care proxy. Her directive reads as follows: "I direct my attending physician to withhold or withdraw treatment that merely prolongs my dying, if I should be in an incurable or irreversible mental or physical condition with no reasonable expectation of recovery, including but not limited to: (a) a terminal condition; (b) a permanently unconscious condition; or (c) a minimally conscious condition in which I am permanently unable to make decisions or express my wishes. I direct that my treatment be limited to measures to keep me comfortable and to relieve pain that might occur by withholding or withdrawing treatment. While I understand that I am not

legally required to be specific about future treatments, if I am in the
conditions described above I feel especially strongly about the following
forms of treatment: I do not want cardiac resuscitation. I do not want
mechanical respiration. I do not want artificial nutrition and hydration.
I do not want antibiotics. However, I do want maximum pain relief,
even if it may hasten my death."

Mrs. Robinson's family and health care providers have been concerned about her diet and nutritional status for years. She always has
eaten small portions and claims to have no appetite. She weighs 94
pounds, which is significantly below her ideal weight range. Nutritional
supplements and medication to increase her appetite have had little
effect. Now, for the past several weeks Mrs. Robinson has been refusing
meals and saying repeatedly, "I'm ready to go home." Her family has
brought in her favorite foods to encourage intake. However, she refuses
to eat and has been refusing medications as well. As she is becoming
increasingly weak, she spends more time in bed. During visits from the
chaplain, Mrs. Robinson was asked directly if she was not eating because
she wanted to die and she replied, "Yes." She has talked about how
overwhelmed she feels and how tired she is. However, it has been
difficult to explore her feelings in greater detail because of her confusion and inability to remain focused. Her daughter flew in to see her,
and all family members are worried and distressed to see Mrs. Robinson
in such physical decline. The son in particular is feeling conflicted as
he struggles between his desire to revitalize his mother and his duty
to see that her advance directives are followed. He believes that the
statement—"I'm ready to go home"—is consistent with his mother's
religious beliefs and means that his mother has actively chosen to end
her earthly life in anticipation of going to her heavenly home. He knows
that his mother would not want him to intervene, but in care conference
he asks staff members for their understanding of the advance directives
and their professional views on what to do in this situation.

Staff members are fond of Mrs. Robinson and distressed by her
refusals of nourishment and medication. She takes only small sips of
water and is becoming more lethargic. Lab values indicate malnutrition
and possible dehydration. There is no evidence of reversible medical
illness that could account for her behavior. Past psychiatric evaluation
had confirmed a depressive syndrome with underlying dementia for
which she was receiving the medication that she will no longer take.
Nursing personnel continue to bring meals to her and offer assistance,
but to no avail. She now requires assistance with all activities of daily
living. She also has had episodes of urinary incontinence. The care
team has advised the family that comfort care is consistent with her

previously expressed wishes and that even now she appears to be maintaining control over her choices. However, they, too, experience feelings of discomfort and helplessness.

Some staff members disagree with the care team's recommendation and ask: (1) Is her current behavior secondary to some unknown/undetected medical or psychiatric condition? (2) Would discharge back to the community with 24-hour care make her happier and encourage her to start eating again? (3) Would her proxy be able to reverse her documented decision to abstain from tube feedings and IV fluids since she now lacks capacity to personally reinforce the conditions of the living will? (4) Is it appropriate to consider her present state as an "incurable or irreversible mental or physical condition with no reasonable expectation of recovery"? (5) How will staff find support for a sense of helplessness in the face of Mrs. Robinson's drastic decline?

Negative Right: Learning the Limits of Intervention

The issue is an individual's right not to receive treatment against his/her expressed wishes.

Dialogue

Where is the *ethical conflict* or dilemma of *competing goods?*

Are there *questions* brought to mind but not answered by the narrative?

Institutional policies: What is the institutional policy on advance directives? What practices and procedures are followed in end-of-life care?

Meaning in resident's actions: To what extent could depression, pain, swallowing difficulties, or ineffective mealtime assistance be a basis for Mrs. Robinson's refusal to eat and expressed wish to die?

The role dementia plays: What are the indicators of being in the terminal phase of life for persons with progressive dementia (e.g., see Rabins et al., 1999, Chapter 9: Terminal Care)?

Related sources: Kayser-Jones & Pengilly (1999). Dysphagia among nursing home residents; Kayser-Jones & Schell (1997b). The mealtime experience of a cognitively impaired elder: Ineffective and effective strategies; Finucane, Christmas, & Travis (1999). Tube feeding in patients with advanced dementia and commentary by McCann (1999); Post (2001). Tube feeding and advanced progressive dementia; Scarpinato, Schell, & Kagan (2000). Kitty's Dilemma: Making treatment decisions when a patient with dementia says she wants to end her life.

What are pros and cons of the following *possible actions*? Are there *other recommendations*?
Possible Actions:

1. Continue to evaluate what Mrs. Robinson is trying to communicate by refusing food and medication.
2. Hold meetings for staff in which they may bring up issues that are bothering them and acknowledge together the discomfort of dealing with situations of this sort.
3. Forward this case to the ethics committee for its recommendations.
4. Discontinue efforts to feed Mrs. Robinson and provide comfort care in accordance with the wishes expressed in her advance directives.
5. Begin tube feedings until the issue is resolved.

Commentary on I'm Ready to Go Home

Ethical Considerations

Ethical principles of providing nurturing care (beneficence) and respecting Mrs. Robinson's wishes (autonomy) are at issue.

Competing Goods Might Be:

It is good to let the resident be in control.
It is good to provide high quality personal care.

It is good to follow a person's advance directives.
It is good to know when to follow a person's advance directives.

It is good to live.
It is good to die, if one's time to die has come.

Questions

How can family and staff be supported, given Mrs. Robinson's drastic decline and their sense of helplessness? To what degree can the resident's words and actions be understood as a clear choice? Are staff and family correctly interpreting her wishes?

Discussion of *pros and cons of "possible actions"* might be as follows:

Possible Action #1

Continue to evaluate the meaning of Mrs. Robinson's refusal of food and medication.

PRO: This action aims to keep open all possible communication pathways between Mrs. Robinson and others and permits further exploration. For example, does she have an undiagnosed swallowing disorder or treatable medical condition? Is she in pain or depressed? Do care practices or environmental factors contribute to her behavior?

Possible Action #2

Hold meetings for staff in which they may bring up issues that are bothering them and acknowledge the discomfort of dealing with situations of this sort.

PRO: This action focuses on listening to and supporting staff members in this difficult situation. Staff members need also to consider how they can work through their own feelings sufficiently to provide needed support to Mrs. Robinson's family.
CON: It may seem like window dressing if no action is taken, frustrating staff further.

Possible Action #3

Forward this case to the ethics committee.

PRO: A committee perspective on the similarities and differences across cases of this type may be helpful. The committee also can be helpful in gathering and stating the facts of the case in a way that may facilitate consensus around the best course of action. Reaching consensus often is difficult even when there are advance directives. (See Hurley, Volicer, Rempusheski, & Fry, 1995—Reaching consensus: The process of recommending treatment decisions for Alzheimer's patients; see also Rempusheski & Hurley, 2000—Advance directives and dementia.) And major obstacles to palliation and end-of-life care are reported to be failure to recognize treatment futility, lack of communication among decision-makers, no agreement on a course for end-of-life care, and failure to implement a timely end-of-life care plan (Travis et al., 2002).

Possible Action #4

Discontinue efforts to feed Mrs. Robinson and provide comfort care in accordance with the wishes expressed in her advance directives.

PRO: This action honors Mrs. Robinson's wishes as expressed in her advance directives. It will lead to a relatively peaceful death in about two or three weeks.
CON: Honoring the advance directives causes pain and discomfort to family and staff members who are charged with carrying out these wishes. There also are the doubts and questions regarding whether or not it is the right time to follow the directives as well as, possibly, fears about legal/regulatory ramifications.

Possible Action #5

Begin tube feedings until the issue is resolved.

PRO: This action is aimed at maintaining physiological function through administration of food and fluid. It addresses whatever doubts there may be about the wisdom of following the advance directives at this time.
CON: Instituting an intervention that Mrs. Robinson previously stated she did not want creates a new situation in which questions will eventually focus on continuing versus ending the tube feedings. It is likely that these discussions will be no less painful than the ones that preceded them. The remaining questions will be whether or not this intervention was justified in the first place and what additional discomfort or distress the procedure itself may have caused, including untoward consequences, such as aspiration pneumonia. Rabins et al. (1999) caution that "there is no single right answer to the questions surrounding feeding tube placement" (p. 246). However, clinical evidence suggests that assisted oral feeding and quality end-of-life care are better options for persons with advanced progressive dementia.

CASE EXAMPLE 11. PLEASE, JUST ONE MORE BITE

Pearl Siebert is a 94-year-old resident of Friendship Villa who, following her husband's death and for six years prior to admission, lived with her only daughter and son-in-law in their home. Her progressive confusion and memory problems made the year before admission particularly challenging for them, and even with the assistance of a paid helper, by the time she came to Friendship Villa, they were "beyond burnout." Mrs. Siebert executed a living will and appointed her daughter as her health care proxy at the time that she came to live with her.

Mrs. Siebert has a history of delusions and behavior changes accompanying her dementia that have been followed by her psychiatrist and have required medications intermittently. Additionally, she is controlled on medication for heart disease, has a chronic sleep disorder, and is legally blind due to cataracts, glaucoma, and macular degeneration. She has some difficulty swallowing and needs to be fed.

On the day of admission, Mrs. Siebert was extremely violent, agitated, striking out, wandering, and uncontrollable. She was oriented to self and recognized her daughter and son-in-law. Medication has reduced the agitation but has caused sedation, increasing her risk for falls and aspiration. Each adjustment of the medication involves a trade-off of a moderate level of sedation in exchange for decreased agitation, wandering, and aggressive behavior toward staff and other residents. The daughter is very distressed by the episodes of agitation and angry over what she observes to be less than total care of her mother when they occur. Her anger and frustration with the nursing home have increased following several falls that have occurred in the process of nursing staff's efforts to deliver care. Mrs. Siebert was lethargic for a period of time after these falls but there was no evidence of injury, and she improved slowly. Her daughter has been told in frequent and repeated conversations that the situation indicates deterioration caused by Mrs. Siebert's disease conditions. Finding the middle ground is exceedingly difficult, because the family is angry and upset when she is either over-sedated or when sedation is reduced and Mrs. Siebert becomes so agitated that adequate care delivery is impossible.

Other residents have been complaining that Mrs. Siebert wanders in and out of their rooms and has been harassing them. There is a physician's order for "a gerichair [chair that restricts movement] prn [as needed] to prevent her from leaving the unit during periods of agitation and excessive wandering." The daughter agreed to this. Shortly thereafter, staff recommended transfer of her mother to the facility's special care unit, which the daughter resisted. She said that she wanted her mother to remain on the unit where she was, in the gerichair, rather than have the freedom to wander on the special care unit. The psychiatrist who has been following Mrs. Siebert for many years observes that the daughter appears to be having difficulty in accepting her mother's behaviors and the deteriorating nature of her illnesses.

Currently, the care team has been meeting with Mrs. Siebert's daughter and son-in-law regarding her occasional refusal of meals and medications. Mrs. Siebert will shove caregivers away when they offer food and attempt to feed her. She resists medication by clenching her teeth or spitting out the medication upon its administration. She also attempts to slap, pinch, scratch, spit, and bite during efforts to bathe, dress, transfer, or toilet her. At these times, she verbally abuses staff and demands that they go away and leave her alone.

The daughter has requested a forceful approach. She reports encountering a nursing assistant who was trying to coax her mother to eat with attempts to entertain and distract her with conversation, stories, and songs. However she was getting nowhere with entreaties of "Please, just one more bite." Mrs. Siebert was spitting out food, pushing the nursing assistant's hand away, and attempting to throw her tray on the floor. The daughter stormed into the office of the Director of Nursing shouting, "How can a woman who is not mentally competent be allowed to dictate what she will and will not do?" At her meeting with the social worker she said, "I want you to know that I've called the Department of Health; and I've been told that my mother has the right to receive food and medications. If she isn't competent, Friendship Villa's responsibility is to follow up on these rights." The social worker provided the daughter with a copy of Friendship Villa's statement of Residents' Rights and explained that the nursing home's policy supports a firm approach, but honors a resident's rights to refuse. Mrs. Siebert's daughter insists that it is impossible for her mother to knowingly exercise such a right due to her confusion.

The daughter has been an extremely active participant in her mother's care. She comes in to feed her most evening meals, sometimes bringing in her favorite foods. Mrs. Siebert does not strike out at her daughter, but she does resist. When she attempts to push food away, her daughter restrains her; when she clenches her teeth, her daughter holds her nose until she opens her mouth; when she refuses to swallow her daughter rubs her throat and repeatedly insists that she "swallow that" until she complies. These mealtimes in her room involve much struggling, loud yelling, and arguing, but Mrs. Siebert's daughter, generally, prevails. And, since she is relatively successful in her efforts, she does not understand why staff members cannot follow suit in her absence. The daughter strongly supports and advocates for her mother in a number of other ways as well. She notes and reports changes in Mrs. Siebert's physical condition; requests eyeglass adjustments; takes her for rides and home visits; brings her snacks; and calls every day to ask how she has been and if there have been any changes. She responds well to staff taking time to listen to her concerns and expresses appreciation of staff assurances that they are doing their best. But she remains angry, believing that "their best is not good enough" and that the nursing home is not doing all that can be done for her mother.

NEGATIVE RIGHT: LEARNING THE LIMITS OF INTERVENTION

The issue is one of Mrs. Siebert's right not to be forced to do things.

Dialogue

Where is the *ethical conflict* or dilemma of *competing goods?*

Are there *questions* brought to mind but not answered by the narrative?

Institutional policies: What are the policies and procedures relating to (a) use of force in caring for residents and (b) a plan to promote workplace safety for staff?

Meaning in resident's actions: What factors may account for Mrs. Siebert's refusals of food, medication, and other forms of care (e.g., fatigue, pain, discomfort, environmental change or distractions, caregiver behavior, fear or delusions)? Is oral hygiene a factor? Does mouth and throat dryness as a side effect of medications make food hard to swallow? Is she fearful of choking? Do changes in taste sensation make some foods unpalatable? Are there discernable food dislikes and preferences? Is food served at the correct temperature and does it appear appetizing?

The role dementia plays: What is Mrs. Siebert's ability to eat? For example, does she chew food for a long time, forget to swallow, not chew food before swallowing, or exhibit other eating difficulties seen in persons at later stages of dementia? Are her delusional symptoms a factor in her occasional refusals of food and medications, that is, does she fear someone is trying to harm her? Has her nutritional status been significantly affected?

Related sources: Durnbaugh, Haley, & Roberts (1996). Assessing problem feeding behaviors in mid-stage Alzheimer's disease; Kayser-Jones & Schell (1997a).The effect of staffing on the quality of care at meal-time; Mahoney et al. (2000). *Management of challenging behaviors in dementia* (Chapter 10—preventing food refusal); Gates, Fitzwater, & Meyer (1999). Violence against caregivers in nursing homes; Horgas & Tsai (1998). Analgesic drug prescription and use in cognitively impaired nursing home residents; Epps (2001). Recognizing pain in the institutionalized elder with dementia.

What are pros and cons of the following *possible actions?* Are there *other recommendations?*

Possible Actions:

1. Mrs. Siebert's daughter may participate in her mother's care as she believes is best; but the family must understand that staff may not force feed the resident because it constitutes abuse.
2. The facility has a responsibility to force care and treatments because residents who lack capacity, or are demented, do not have the "right" to refuse.
3. The facility's first responsibility is to follow the wishes of the daughter in her role as Mrs. Siebert's health care proxy.
4. Continue close communication with Mrs. Siebert's daughter, encouraging her to think things through and helping her anticipate care issues and treatment plans.

Commentary on Please, Just One More Bite

Ethical Considerations

Ethical principles involving resident rights (autonomy) and provision of basic care (beneficence) are at issue. Mrs. Siebert needs to receive nourishment and medication. She also has the right to refuse care. The disagreement concerns whether or not her dementia justifies disregarding her rights and, if not, there is the question of how to determine when the line between meeting her needs and violating her rights has been crossed. An additional issue concerns the appropriateness of allowing Mrs. Siebert to remain where she is versus transfer to the special care unit. What is fair (justice) in meeting her needs versus the needs of other residents?

Competing Goods Might Be:

It is good to incorporate resident and family wishes into the plan of care.
It is good to follow a plan of care based on professional judgment and facility policies.

It is good for a resident to remain in a familiar environment.
It is good for residents to live on a unit where other residents are not disturbed.

Questions

What is the nursing home's policy concerning use of force to deliver care? Is there a difference between the daughter's use of force in feeding her mother and the same use of force by staff members?

Is staffing adequate for taking needed time and using best approaches for assisting residents at mealtime?

What policies and practices are in place for promoting workplace safety? Do caregivers receive special training in preventing and managing physical and verbal abuse from residents and other people?

Could undiagnosed pain partially explain Mrs. Siebert's behavior?

Would more staff member contact with the daughter and son-in-law be helpful? Would a support group be helpful to the family?

Do nursing home personnel need support in dealing with family member stress? Family members may redirect their emotional burdens of frustration, grief, fear, guilt, or anger over what is happening to their loved ones and themselves by "taking out their feelings on nursing home administrators and staff. [This reaction may take the form of] blaming, badgering, or inappropriately accusing people who work [at the nursing home over matters pertaining to] their relative's treatment. [Family members who do this] may not even be conscious of their motives and feel they are acting as advocates; but it leaves staff with the dilemma of how to respond to people who are confronting them in these presumably unjustified but emotionally understandable ways" (J. Savishinsky, personal communication, June 4, 2002). This situation itself is another example of an everyday ethical issue.

Discussion of *pros and cons of "possible actions"* might be as follows:

Possible Action #1

Mrs. Siebert's daughter may participate in her mother's care as she believes is best, but the family must understand that staff may not force-feed the resident because that would constitute abuse.

PRO: This action supports Mrs. Siebert's right to refuse and protects her from what may be viewed as abuse by staff.

CON: It leaves open the debate concerning what constitutes abuse. Specifically, it raises the question of whether or not the facility is supporting a form of abuse by allowing the daughter to force-feed her mother.

Possible Action #2

The facility has a responsibility to force care and treatments because residents who lack capacity, or are demented, do not have the "right" to refuse.

PRO: This position suggests a need to compensate for residents with diminished capacity to make their own decisions by making some decisions for them and being sure that they comply with what is judged to be in their best interests.
CON: It does not take into consideration the fact that residents with dementia do at times have an understanding of situations that would enable them to knowingly exercise their rights. As an unconditional statement, it is paternalistic, disrespectful, and untrue.

Possible Action #3

The facility's first responsibility is to follow the wishes of the daughter in her role as Mrs. Siebert's health care proxy.

PRO: This position supports the importance of working collaboratively with those who have been designated as residents' health care proxies.
CON: It does not allow for questioning whether or not the daughter is exceeding her role as proxy. The nursing home's primary responsibility is to Mrs. Siebert. Therefore, some consensus needs to be reached regarding how closely the daughter's wishes reflect how her mother ordinarily would have wished to be treated under these circumstances. Resolving the issue of which nursing home unit best fits her current needs is another area where the judgment of nursing home staff should be considered along with the daughter's wishes.

Possible Action #4

Continue close communication with Mrs. Siebert's daughter, encouraging her to think things through and helping her anticipate care issues and treatment plans.

PRO: This action emphasizes the daughter's need for help and support in a stressful situation. The grief and guilt that families experience in having to place loved ones in a nursing home and then watching them decline is enormous. It will help to view their actions in that context and to provide ample time to listen to them and to reassure them through being readily available and by taking the initiative for frequent and regular contact.

To "Let Go" Takes Love

To "let go" is not to cut myself off,
     it is the realization I can't control another.

To "let go" is not to enable,
     but to allow learning from natural consequences.

To "let go" is to admit powerlessness,
     which means the outcome is not in my hands.

To "let go" is not to try to change or blame another,
     it is to make the most of myself.

To "let go" is not to care for, but to care about.

To "let go" is not to fix, but to be supportive.

To "let go" is not to judge, but to allow another to be a human being.

To "let go" is not to be in the middle arranging all the outcomes
     but to allow others to affect their own destinies.

To "let go" is not to be protective,
     it is to permit another to face reality.

To "let" go is not to deny, but to accept.

To "let go" is not to nag, scold, or argue, but instead
     to search out my own shortcomings and to correct them.

To "let go" is not to adjust everything to my desires
     but to take each day as it comes, and cherish myself in it.

To "let go" is not to criticize and regulate anybody
     but to try to become what I dream I can be.

To "let go" is to not regret the past,
     but to grow and to live for the future.

To "let go" is to fear less and to love more.

FIGURE 4.1   To "let go" takes love.

Originally published by Sr. Anne Maloy, Sr. M. Gratia L'Esperance, & Mrs. Lucia Zerón-Castillejo (Eds.) in *Resource Guide for Planning the Care of Aged Loved Ones*, ©2002, p. 50. Used with the permission of Mercy Center with the Aging, Rochester, New York.

CON: It is a approach that does not immediately resolve the short-term issues over residents' rights or the daughter's concerns about her mother receiving food and medications. But it takes them into account by recognizing larger issues in which these concerns may be embedded, that is, issues related to family members' anguish, fear, and suffering. The following thoughts illustrate what this experience may be like.

> This seemingly unresolvable situation is one through which most families and staff eventually will have to pass. It reflects the struggle and pain of relinquishing control of the uncontrollable that dementia brings to our lives. It is a dilemma for which there seems to be no easy solution. But in a passage written by The Mercy Center with the Aging in Rochester, NY a new perspective may be found. This writing takes on additional meaning when it is realized that the underlining of the passage shown here was made by a woman in the early to middle stages of dementia. It was her lifelong habit to underline those words that had special meaning to her. So her strong but unsteady hand seems to suggest that *these words* resonate deeply with her, personally, about *her own* struggle to let go and that, through her underlining, she also may have communicated something to her family—giving them—at some future time—permission to let go of her, with love. (Confidential personal communication, used with permission, July 2, 2002)

The above referred to reflection *"To 'Let Go' Takes Love"* is reprinted with permission from the Mercy Center with the Aging in Rochester, New York. It is believed that its message applies equally to residents, families, and staff.

CASE EXAMPLE 12. GET ME OUT OF HERE

Bert Van Buren is a 92-year-old man who was admitted to Colonie Manor 18 months ago following hospitalization for a left hip fracture. His medical history includes degenerative arthritis and dementia, likely of the Alzheimer's type, with intermittent forgetfulness and a balance deficit. His post-surgical rehabilitation was successful and he progressed to full weight bearing without significant pain. Following rehabilitation, he was able to walk with a walker and standby assistance. His gait was stable with no significant weakness. Over the last six months, his forgetfulness has worsened and his attention span is less than it had been. He is unable to recall events of 5–30 minutes prior on repeated questioning. He fell when getting out of his wheelchair, and, while x-rays showed no evidence of a fracture of the surgical hip, he did have a pelvic fracture that was treated with bed rest and non-weight bearing for a few weeks followed by aggressive therapy. In two months he was able to bear weight, and orthopedic evaluation showed good healing of the pelvic fracture. Thus, full ambulation now is allowed.

At this point the family is strongly united in their request that Mr. Van Buren be restrained at all times to protect him from the possibility of future falls. Mr. Van Buren repeatedly has tried to get out of bed and the wheelchair by himself. And medical orders have been written for the use of a soft safety device while in bed and a rollbar for safety while in the wheelchair. However, he has been very agitated with the restraints. He removed the rollbar and a waist restraint was applied. He struggled to get out of every kind of restraint, calling out loudly, "Get me out of here! Get me out of here!" He tells family members, "I would like to cut these off. I hate being tied up." But they insist that restraints are necessary and tell him, "You need to have these so you won't fall again and break something." A number of times, nursing home staff have tried to leave him unrestrained during the day when he can be monitored. However, he gets up from his chair quickly and does not remember to use the walker. Consequently, restraints were reapplied pending further evaluation.

Colonie Manor has a restraint minimization policy, and staff would like to accommodate Mr. Van Buren's desire to be unrestrained as much as possible. The care team has discussed quality of life issues with the family and described Mr. Van Buren's distressed reactions to restraints as indicative of a need to consider continuation of attempts to limit their use. He was reported to be spending all of his time and energy trying to get out of the chair restraints. And he was trying to jump out of bed with the rails up to avoid setting off the bed alarm. There is a written order that says "may remove restraint when visitors are present," but the family believes that Mr. Van Buren is more upset and agitated when restraints need to be reapplied than he would be if they simply became a permanent part of his treatment plan. Meanwhile, Mr. Van Buren has gained a reputation for being highly successful at removing and struggling out of restraints. When he could not escape, he would twist and knot restraints in ways that had the potential to cause injury. Staff have started a flow sheet to document all restraint-related activity and the Director of Social Work has discussed the Health Department Code, institutional restraint minimization policy, and "liability potential" with the Colonie Manor attorney.

Members of the care team do not agree on the best course of action to take. Some staff members think that the family's insistence is a good reason not to "rock the boat." They suggest that: "He's not complaining as much anymore; he really is too confused, and you know he would fall; now that the vest restraint is tied behind his back, he can't get to it as easily; and we don't have the resources to provide 1:1 care if he's not restrained."

At the quarterly care planning meeting, however, the social worker and nurse manager proposed a trial restraint removal five times a day for 30 minutes with 1:1 supervision by nursing and social work to assess Mr.Van Buren's reaction to being unrestrained and to prevent unassisted ambulation and falls. The family at first agreed to the plan, despite their restated fear of falls. However, later they individually called the social worker to say that they had changed their minds and were adamantly against Colonie Manor removing the restraints. They followed up with a letter repeating the importance of continued use of restraints for Mr.Van Buren's safety and well being and copied it to their attorney. The team decided that the trial would not proceed. Mr.Van Buren, meanwhile, is quieter and struggling less, although he tells the social worker and staff involved in applying the restraints, "I really hate what you're doing to me . . . I feel like a dirty dog tied up like this . . . You treat me like a dog . . . But my family says I have to have it [the restraint]. It keeps me safe, and they know what's best for me."

NEGATIVE RIGHT: TEMPERING THE CULTURE OF SURVEILLANCE AND RESTRAINT

The issue is one of individual rights not to be restrained, confined, or intruded upon. Personal integrity also is threatened by loss of dignity. An additional organizational-level issue is one of personnel resources.

Dialogue

Where is the *ethical conflict* or dilemma of *competing goods*?

Are there *questions* brought to mind but not answered by the narrative?

Institutional policies: What are the policies on Residents' Rights and use of physical and chemical restraints? What policies and procedures are to be followed in the event that a resident falls? What reports and documentation are required?

Meaning in resident's actions: How do restraints affect Mr. Van Buren's dignity? What further motivates him to struggle against them? How can physical restraints cause, rather than prevent, injury?

The role dementia plays: What level of supervision does Mr. Van Buren need to protect him from harm? How may use/nonuse of the restraints make a difference in reduction of falls? Cognitive impairment is not sufficient reason for restraint. Has a recent falls risk assessment been done?

Related sources: Collopy (1992). The use of restraints in long-term care: The ethical issues (American Association of Homes for the Aging White Paper); American Geriatrics Society, British Geriatric Society & American Academy of Orthopaedic Surgeons Panel on Falls Prevention (2001). Guideline for the prevention of falls in older persons; Rubenstein (2000). Approaching falls in older persons; Strumpf, Robinson, Wagner, & Evans (1998). Restraint-free care.

What are pros and cons of the following *possible actions*? Are there *other recommendations*?

Possible Actions:

1. Educate the family about the limits of restraints—that they cannot always prevent falls and can in themselves present significant risk of injury. Thus, they do not offer absolute protection from physical harm. And, at the same time, they introduce the possibility of causing emotional harm to residents who may express distress, fear, outrage, and/or humiliation at being treated this way. If restraint is deemed a necessary protection, the least restrictive means should be used.
2. Reassess use of restraints for Mr. Van Buren quarterly, or sooner if he has complaints.
3. Continue use of restraints in accordance with family wishes.
4. Educate facility staff about issues associated with restraint-free/independence promoting practices.

Commentary on Get Me Out of Here

Ethical Considerations

Ethical principles of personal freedom (autonomy) and doing good and preventing harm (beneficence) are at issue. For family members, the desire to prevent harm to Mr. Van Buren overrides his desire for independence and freedom from the restraints.

Competing Goods Might Be:

It is good to decrease falls versus it is good to be free of restraint.

It is good to support resident independence versus it is good to support family wishes.

It is good to increase resident well-being versus it is good to support family well-being.

It is good to have care provider consensus versus it is good to have team member individuality.

It is good to decrease use of restraints versus it is good not to be sued.

It is good to follow policies and meet regulations versus it is good not to cause conflict.

Questions

We know nothing about what sort of person Mr. Van Buren was prior to his admission. Was he a very active person? How does being tied to a chair for hours at a time compare to the manner of life he used to lead? Are there appropriate activities in which he might be engaged that might distract attention from the restraints or reduce reliance on them?

We know nothing about family relationships beyond members' united stand against removing Mr. Van Buren's restraints. Does someone have health care proxy? What is the entire scope of family concerns surrounding Mr. Van Buren and his care? How do family members communicate with staff and with each other regarding Mr. Van Buren's needs?

What are the staffing issues that limit monitoring Mr. Van Buren more closely?

Discussion of *pros and cons of "possible actions"* might be:

Possible Action #1

Educate the family about the limits of restraints—that they cannot always prevent falls and can in themselves present significant risk of injury. Thus, they do not offer absolute protection from physical harm. And, at the same time, they introduce the possibility of causing emotional harm to residents who may express distress, fear, outrage and/or humiliation at being treated this way. If restraint is deemed a necessary protection, the least restrictive means should be used.

PRO: This action seeks to inform family members about the use of restraints and the reasons that support a restraint minimization policy. Discussion should include Mr. Van Buren's history of falls with a careful evaluation of their frequency and surrounding circumstances.

CON: Education requires learner interest and time. Failing to engage family members in a positive way or rushing the process may yield negative results.

Possible Action #2

Reassess use of restraints for Mr. Van Buren quarterly, or sooner if he voices complaints.

PRO: This action keeps the matter open to continuous and systematic review. It also allows Mr. Van Buren to activate the reassessment process through voicing complaints. A comprehensive assessment may identify falls risk factors that are modifiable through gait, balance, and exercise programs; adjustment of medications; treatment for medical conditions such as postural hypotension or cardiovascular disease; correction of vision problems; training on proper use of the walker; or environmental changes to reduce hazards and increase observation/supervision. Hip protectors, though not reducing risk of falls, also may lower risk of hip fractures in high-risk individuals (American Geriatrics Society et al., 2001).
CON: It does not immediately change the status quo unless modifiable risk factors are found and reduced.

Possible Action #3

Continue use of restraints in accordance with family wishes.

PRO: This action reduces strain on the family around this issue and allays their fears.
CON: But, it increases strain on Mr. Van Buren and has a negative affect on his well-being.

Possible Action #4

Educate facility staff about issues associated with restraint-free/independence promoting practices.

PRO: This action promotes a consistent informed approach to the matter by all facility staff. It has positive implications that affect and reach beyond this individual case.
CON: It will not produce consensus unless there is an effort to listen in an open nonjudgmental way to individual points of view, especially

the views of nursing assistants who provide the actual hands-on care. Staffing issues, in particular, should be carefully evaluated, since they should not be the reason for providing a less than optimum level of supervision.

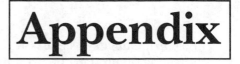

Appendix

Nursing Home Ethics Committee Q & A

Ideas about the **why, where, what, who,** and **how** of a nursing home ethics committee will need to be tailored to the special character and organizational culture of each facility. This chapter addresses the following questions that may be asked initially.

1. Why do we need another committee?
    What are specific needs that could be met by an ethics committee?
2. Where in the organization does the committee fit?
    Whose responsibility is it?
3. What is the primary purpose of the ethics committee?
    What are its usual functions?
4. Who should be represented on the committee?
    How big should the committee be?
5. How is the work of the committee managed?
    How are issues and cases brought forward?
    What processes and procedures are followed?

The last question addressed in this chapter—**Now what?**—is about ongoing appraisal of a committee's work, since it is not unusual for established committees to wonder about their progress or to feel that they need to be reenergized.

WHY DO WE NEED ANOTHER COMMITTEE?

"We deal with these issues all the time. We're so used to dealing with them, I'm not sure that we stop often enough to really think about them."

This staff member's insight is repeated here because it captures a certain feeling about daily life in a nursing home. So, *what is it like to work in a nursing home?* Certified nursing assistants speak about the physical and psychological demands of the job.

> *"It can be stressful sometimes. Sometimes [Mr. X] stresses me out because he's so heavy. You need two people when you're dressing and turning him; and when he resists . . . Oh, boy! You gotta like what you're doing, and you gotta have a lot of patience to do it."*

> *"If you don't want to do it, you're not going to last, because you get mental abuse, verbal abuse, and physical abuse [from residents] and you've got a lot, a lot, a lot to do. This is not an easy job."*

But the demands, difficulties and frustrations of the work represent only one side of the story. Below, nursing assistants tell about personal rewards and emotional ties with residents that also describe what it is like to work in a nursing home.

> *"I like the job. I like to joke with my residents. A lot of them have a great sense of humor. [Mrs. Y] is like a grandmother to me."*

> *"Sometimes I get too attached. I just lost one of my ladies . . . [Mrs. Z] . . . I really loved her. Now, it's okay to get attached; but the really difficult thing is when they pass on."*

Therefore, the "issues we deal with all the time" take into account both sides of the story—the challenges and the rewards of working in a nursing home.

And, *what are these issues we deal with all the time?* In terms of persons with dementia, often there is a continuation of issues that family members have experienced prior to admission to the nursing home, such as the following.

> *Daughter:* *"She lost her watch. And then a couple of other things . . . Of course, I thought that everybody was stealing from her. At that point, I hadn't realized how much people [with dementia] lose things."*

> *Son:* *"She would take the water, and she would take the pills in her hand; but she wouldn't swallow them. And, then she would hide them. We'd find pills all over the house."*

Differences between a home environment and communal life in nursing homes bring out additional issues. Family comments exemplify these new concerns.

Wife: "*Wandering was a big problem. That was a no-no, which I can understand. He got into a lady's room and was going through the drawers. They found him with this little article of clothing, and they said, '[Mr. Q], this isn't your room; and this isn't yours.' And he just smiled and said, 'I thought this looked a little small.' He's got a cute way about him; [but the lady] was really upset.*"

Sister: "*They say they take her down to things [activities/programs] and that she's participating more, but she won't stay. I brought her back [to a program] and she was fine. She enjoyed it. I think if it was one of the aides [sitting next to her], she would be all right. [But], it would have to be someone that she was familiar with.*"

Daughter: "*His first roommate was a very small, frail man. And he used to cover him up, put a pillow on his head, and then, sometimes, he would get in bed with him. So they put him in with a gentleman that was a big guy. They felt that Dad would be pushed away . . . but he wouldn't be hurt. Now he has a new roommate . . . I guess that's working out. I don't know. Sometimes it seems like he doesn't realize he has a roommate.*"

The comment—"*we're so used to dealing with them [everyday issues]*"—refers to examples like the above. "Every resident is different; but, in some ways, every resident is the same," explains one nursing assistant. For staff, the day after day sameness of resident care is in the similarity of human needs for care and nurturing, kindness, and companionship. The differences are as numerous as the individuals themselves. But the repetitive nature of resident care ensures that concerns about one situation will remind caregivers of similar ones. Trying out and analyzing the effectiveness of different approaches to common caregiving challenges becomes a taken for granted activity. Over time, staff hesitate less and become more successful at resolving everyday issues through a combination of expertise and intuition—or, in the words of our above quoted staff member, "*without stopping to really think about them.*"

And what does it mean to "*deal with issues all the time without stopping to really think about them?*" Familiarity with common issues and being used to dealing with them accounts for the natural ease with which some individuals and groups (unit staff/resident care teams) reach decisions about the best way to solve problems and address concerns.

Of course people are thinking about the issues. It is their awareness of not being able to stop for long that creates a sense of not stopping "*often enough.*" The circumstances that keep us moving without stopping include the urgency of things that require immediate attention, the stress of competing demands, physical and emotional fatigue, and the limits of time. We all have these experiences. The regret of not stopping often enough to sort out concerns, troubles, and annoyances as they come up again and again is the sure knowledge that the issues are repetitive ones that will not go away. But, to "*really think*" about an issue is to stop and take the time:

(a) To go over and over details of the contexts in which it arises;

(b) To ask questions that lead to deeper more complete understanding of what it is all about from the resident's point of view;

(c) To view it from different perspectives;

(d) To seek out additional information;

(e) To identify and explore differences of opinion;

(f) To weigh alternative courses of action; and

(g) To acknowledge personal values and biases that may influence choices and preferences regarding how it ought to be resolved.

If we were always thinking this deeply and intensely about what is happening while it is happening, our work would never get done.

So, *why do we need another committee?* This is a good question, particularly for people with a sense of little enough time to stop already. It may help to think about it, not in terms of taking time, but in terms of creating a place to go—moral space in which ethical thinking unfolds. An ethics committee provides space for *"really thinking"* in a reflective, respectful manner about issues that affect residents, families, and nursing home staff. It is not a substitute for individual initiatives and team approaches to care. But it can be a helpful resource to individuals, teams, and the nursing home community.

WHAT ARE SPECIFIC NEEDS THAT COULD BE MET BY AN ETHICS COMMITTEE?

Hospital ethics committees have a long history of responding to situations involving difficult life-and-death choices, such as discontinuing artificial life-support systems and terminating or withholding treatment that would be futile and merely prolong dying. Nursing home ethics committees have a more recent history. They also deal with end-of-life issues that typically involve questions about residents' previously expressed wishes and current competence to make autonomous choices versus others' (family, surrogate, and staff) judgments about what would be in their best interests such as:

When is it time to honor advance directives? Advance directives are specific about the circumstances under which aggressive measures to prolong life should cease. But it is not always easy for caregivers to know when that point has been reached.

What measures promote comfort vs. prolong life? Education about palliative (comfort) care is needed. It is a difficult ethical choice for family and caregivers to withhold or withdraw artificial means of life support such as feeding tubes or intravenous hydration, even in the presence of advance directives. Ability of treatment (e.g., antibiotics) to ease discomfort vs. prolong life may be debated. And decisions to hospitalize to increase comfort/relieve pain vs. use of hospitalization that unduly prolongs life is another aspect of these kinds of discussions.

What measures relieve pain vs. hasten death? Education is needed to better assess residents' pain and address others' fears about actively hastening death by following pain relief protocols involving powerful drugs.

Who decides? Competency and ability of the resident to decide what should be done is the first concern. Substituted judgments must be made if the resident is unable to actively participate. Families and caregivers may experience discomfort in carrying out wishes of a person that have been dictated far in advance of circumstances that call for the directives to be carried out. Family members may disagree among themselves. Surrogates may experience uncertainty about a resident's wishes. Opinions of staff and family/surrogate wishes may differ. And, in the absence of family or other designated surrogate, nursing home staff may be uncertain about the wishes/best interests of unresponsive/questionably competent residents.

In contrast to the illness focus of hospital ethics cases and acute care/end-of-life nursing home cases, there are many more opportunities in nursing homes to investigate concerns about issues of daily living. This normative ethics focus involves values about what it means to "have a good life." Ethical problems occur when values conflict. Examples of conflicting values, expressed in terms of competing goods (e.g., inherently good principles that cannot both be satisfied in a particular circumstance) might be:

Resident refusal of care: It is good to let the resident be in control versus it is good to provide high quality care that meets mandated standards. It is good to have the right to refuse care versus it is good for caregivers to be safe and not in physical danger when giving needed care.

Roommate difficulties: It is good to have privacy and personal space versus it is good to have a friendly relationship and share limited space. It is good to live one's life as one wishes versus it is good to treat others with courtesy and consideration (e.g., lights on/off, noise/sound levels, room too hot/too cold, non-synchronized routines, interruptions, rudeness, idiosyncratic behaviors, invasion of privacy/personal space, disturbance of personal property are common issues). It is good to care for one's roommate versus it is good not to feel responsible for the care of one's roommate.

Married couples: It is good for married couples to room together/ assist each other versus it is good for individual needs for care/ safety/dignity/personal respect to be met through the assistance of staff.

Intimate (nonmarital) relationships: It is good to support individual values and needs for intimacy versus it is good to avoid individual exploitation/hurting others/offending community values about expressions of intimacy.

Married/close friendship relationships: It is good to spend time together/ care for one another versus it is good to engage in individual activities/receive needed individual care. It is good to let couples/friends resolve their own differences versus it is good for others not to be adversely affected by their conflict.

Surveillance and restraint: It is good to maintain privacy versus it is good to promote individual safety. It is good to encourage maximum activity as the resident wishes versus it is good to prevent falls/support family wishes.

Individualized routines: It is good to have a routine/schedule tailored to meet individual needs versus it is good to have routines/schedules that enable the facility to effectively meet residents' group needs.

In-house relocations: It is good for the resident to remain in a familiar setting versus it is good to meet special needs/respect the rights of other residents. "Aging in place" is good versus it is good for residents to be where the level of care that they need can be best delivered.

Conflicts among residents: It is good for a resident to make choices and to socialize versus it is good to protect and respect feelings of other residents. It is good for the resident to have the right to use public space and property (e.g., sitting areas and furnishings) versus it is good for others in the area not to be verbally/physically intimidated (i.e., territoriality). It is good for small groups to have the right to use common space versus it is good for larger groups to have the right to use common space.

Socially unacceptable behaviors: It is good for residents to have freedom of movement and choice/opportunities for socialization versus it is good to protect other residents, families, and visitors from disturbing, inappropriate resident behaviors. It is good to accept idiosyncratic behavior versus it is good to protect the dignity of the resident him/herself from behavior that at one time he/she would have found embarrassing and humiliating.

Truth telling: Telling the truth/not keeping secrets is good versus not hurting others' feelings/avoiding conflicts is good.

Resident withdrawal from others/refusal to socialize: It is good for the resident to have the right to be by him/herself vs. it is good to prevent loneliness/isolation. It is good for the resident to have the right to refuse socialization vs. it is good for the resident to have a social life.

Although all human interactions have value-driven moral aspects, *not all care dilemmas are ethical dilemmas.* Sometimes, communication about an issue results in agreement about the best way to approach it. For example, if a nursing assistant discovers that a resident is less combative and more responsive to assistance with personal care at a certain time of day and reaches consensus with other staff members about the best timing of care activities, the issue revolves around communication. If the care situation generates questions about forcing or manipulating the resident into complying with or conforming to a plan of care, or if there are concerns about fairness to other residents, these would be examples of ethical issues that might benefit from closer examination.

Similarly, a nursing assistant who questions or disagrees with a resident's plan of care may be able to successfully resolve the matter through communication with other staff members. But if the nursing assistant is unsuccessful in raising concerns or goes along with the plan of care despite personal misgivings, this is an ethical dilemma because he/she is being expected to do something that conflicts with what he/she believes is right, good, or fair.

There are many examples of care dilemmas that are resolved successfully by staff members making use of trial and error, knowledge of what has worked in past situations, consensus of opinion, and expert consultation. And there are no rules about what needs to be referred for ethics committee review. This is a matter to be decided by individual facilities and committees in the formation of the official charge and statements of mission and functions. Generally, these committees serve as a resource for resolution of resident issues in morally responsible ways and are not decision-making bodies.

WHERE IN THE ORGANIZATION DOES THE COMMITTEE FIT?

Although the idea of having an ethics committee could come from anywhere in an organization, official support for its establishment and maintenance is desirable. The board of directors or nursing home administrators could sponsor committee formation and determine its official charge and reporting responsibilities within the existing organizational structure. For example, a committee's official charge might be: to provide consultation to staff members in difficult cases; to support a positive ethical climate for residents, families/friends, and staff; to educate itself and the nursing home community about ethical issues; to review, recommend, or develop policies; and to participate in activities related to ethical issues in resident care as a public service.

WHOSE RESPONSIBILITY IS IT?

Ethics committees can be staff committees or administrative committees where leadership and membership more typically follow the management style and bureaucratic structure of the institution. The third type of committee is a board committee that has reporting responsibilities either directly to a facility's board of directors or indirectly to the board through an administrator or another established board committee. This example of high-level support for a committee is advantageous because it communicates that ethical concerns are a serious priority. Its disassociation from management or dominance by any discipline also suggests that members of the committee will have equal status, with each bringing a special type of expertise to bear on issues that are forwarded for review. Thus, it may serve as a model of interdisciplinary collaboration crafted along democratic lines. And it may more visibly indicate a readiness to invite issues on any topic and emanating from any source within the organization.

WHAT IS THE PRIMARY PURPOSE OF THE ETHICS COMMITTEE?

The primary purpose of a nursing home ethics committee is to serve and protect the interests of residents. This consultative role is its most central mission in promoting ethically directed resident care and services. In an advisory capacity, it may make recommendations at the request of anyone, including residents and their families, as long as the concerns are related to this purpose. The facility will need to communicate the appropriate mechanisms for bringing cases forward.

WHAT ARE ITS USUAL FUNCTIONS?

Ethics committees have three major functions: (1) case review; (2) education; and (3) policy review. The amount of time and effort spent on each function may vary from facility to facility and an individual facility also may vary its emphasis across time. Ongoing evaluation of needs will help to determine the appropriate balance of functions.

Case Review

A committee's role in case review should be one of giving informed advice based on investigation of the details of a situation, discussion, and consensus. This is a nonauthoritarian approach that does not imply an obligation on anyone's part to accept the committee's recommendations. However, it should be expected that the committee's contributions will be considered seriously by those responsible for making decisions.

The "ethics facilitation approach" described by ASBH, the American Society for Bioethics and Humanities (1998) has two core features that are applicable to this complex process. The first core feature is *identifying and analyzing the nature of the value uncertainty* through gathering relevant data, clarifying relevant concepts (e.g., privacy, autonomy, best interest, etc.) and normative issues (e.g., implications of law, institutional policy, social values, etc.) and identifying a range of morally acceptable options. The taxonomy framework (Powers, 2001) and the clinical ethics framework (Jonsen et al., 1998) described in Chapter 3 offer ways to structure this activity. However, committees are urged to think about what structure works best for them. Creativity should be encouraged. Committees may borrow elements from more than one approach. There are many ways to organize information. For example, a blending of the two frameworks discussed in Chapter 3 could guide case analysis activity by identifying:

- Ethical Issues
  What are the concerns? Who is affected? What is the resident's condition? What is the plan of care? How does the plan benefit and avoid harm to the resident?
  The nature of the value uncertainty or conflict may be most related to:

  Individual Values
  Learning the limits of interventions (residents' negative rights)
  Preserving individual integrity (residents' positive rights)

  Social Values
  Tempering the culture of surveillance and restraint (residents' negative rights)
  Defining community norms and values (residents' positive rights)

  Clarification of relevant concepts and normative issues occurs through:
  Examining institutional policies (i.e., formal positions and unwritten practices)
  Searching for meaning in residents' actions (i.e., the resident's point of view)
  Evaluating the role dementia plays (i.e., negation of assumptions/ stereotypes)
  Consulting related sources (i.e., credible resources to support deliberation)
- Resident Preferences
  What preferences have been expressed? Are there expressed prior preferences? Who is the designated surrogate? Has the resident/family been informed of the resident's rights, responsibilities, and plan of care? What is the resident's decisional capacity/ legal competency? Is the resident's right to choice and self-determination being respected, ethically and legally?

- Quality of Life
  The resident's view? View of other persons? How is the plan of care expected to improve or maintain the resident's quality of life? Are there any plans to forego treatment? What plans are in place for comfort/palliative care?
- Contextual Features
  What resident-related factors (e.g., personal history; social, economic, religious, cultural variables) may influence recommendations? What institutional factors (e.g., allocation of resources, staffing, work patterns, policies, administration, physical/ social environment) may influence recommendations?

The second ASBH core feature of the ethics facilitation approach is *facilitating the building of consensus* among involved parties (e.g., residents, families, surrogates, staff). This means that ethics committees will need to be sure that everyone's voice is heard and that deliberation includes opportunities for individuals on the committee and those involved in the cases to clarify their own values in a process that leads to building shared understandings about morally acceptable recommendations.

Case review and consultation demands diligence, patience, and a willingness to accept less than perfect solutions. There seldom are perfect solutions to life situations that involve difficult circumstances, strong emotions, and the entangled interests of multiple players. Therefore, in the performance of this committee function, tolerance of ambiguity and a sense of proportion regarding its own limitations are important qualities to foster.

Education

An ethics committee should function to educate itself, members of the nursing home community, and others. *Committee self-education* is a fundamental aspect of its work. Books, articles and reports, case studies (hypothetical and actual current or retrospective cases), and audiovisual material can be used to focus discussion. Colleagues and consultants may give presentations on selected topics.

Orientation sessions should occur when a new committee is formed and be repeated regularly over time as new members are brought in. New members need to understand the committee's mission and procedures, the kinds of issues with which it concerns itself, and the process of ethical deliberation it uses in case review. Some members will need additional orientation to the nursing home community. And everyone, including nursing home staff, will benefit from open discussion about everyday experiences and the additional challenges that dementia brings to the care of a large proportion of the resident population. A committee may decide that it would be more efficient to have individualized or small group orientation for incoming members. Whether done as a whole committee or on an individualized/ small group level, participants should be given written materials in advance with the understanding that they will read and come to orientation sessions prepared to discuss and ask questions.

Regular written *self-evaluations* help committees to assess their progress and set priorities for future work. Types of issues the committee has dealt with will provide information about what the thinking has been on recurring concerns, how cases have been resolved, what topics merit more exploration, where more education is needed, and whether there is a need to recommend additional policies or guidelines. A sense of where a committee has been and where it is going also will provide ideas for conducting ongoing orientation of new members.

Finally, *individual self-education* should be an expectation of all committee members. This can be accomplished by reading relevant books and articles; visiting web sites; attending conferences and seminars; taking a course; or participating in a workshop. Keeping each other informed about discoveries, experiences, and educational opportunities enriches the work of the committee. Sample sources of information and insights are listed at the end of the chapter.

Responsibility for *in-house and wider community education* can be met in a variety of ways. Within its own facility, the committee might, for example:

(a) Develop a collection of books, articles, videos or other subject matter that provides information and supports discussion of ethical issues.

(b) Use existing staff, family, and/or community newsletters and forums to highlight ethical issues.

(c) Start a newsletter focused on ethical issues and solicit reader input and feedback.

(d) Collaborate with the in-service department on educational offerings related to ethical issues.

A committee may not feel that it can provide a wider outreach beyond its own walls. However, it may want to consider visiting, consulting, and benchmarking with other nursing home ethics committees. Ethics committee networks and regional programs provide other kinds of education/dissemination opportunities such as workshops, information and interactive web sites, shared educational materials, and consultation. The possibility of joint sponsorship of seminars or workshops with other local nursing homes also might be explored.

Policy Review

The extent and nature of an ethics committee's involvement in policy matters depends on its charge. Being informed about existing policies is part of its role and it may be asked to offer opinions on policies that are being developed by administrators or governing bodies. Carrying out its case review function also may lead a committee to make recommendations, since this process serves to enhance committee members' awareness of the kinds of issues that would benefit from a new or revised policy. Overall, however, ethics committees are more likely to review and recommend policies than to write them. Knowing what is expected and what the committee is authorized to do in regard to policy is important.

If writing policies is part of its charge, it should be able to draw on legal and administrative counsel from within its own membership, receive appropriate instruction on the formal requirements of policy writing, and clarify the nursing home's procedures for review and acceptance of policies. If there is a separate policy review committee, it might be useful for the ethics committee chair to be a member to facilitate the flow of communication.

Policy writing involves selectivity, since only the most serious, complex, and/or frequently recurring issues will require this type of statement. Policies are not the same as guidelines, the latter being more like suggestions that may be followed at an individual's discretion. Policies are mandatory, and although they may allow room for discretionary actions under certain circumstances, adherence to them is a clear expectation. Nursing homes might be expected to have policies about resident rights and responsibilities; use of force to administer care and treatment; use of physical and chemical restraints; and matters dealing with advance directives, health care proxies/surrogates, and treatment preference options (e.g., comfort care only versus full care, involving all treatments and tests for diagnostic purposes, with or without cardiopulmonary resuscitation).

Committees are responsible for writing their own policies and procedures related to their official charge and reporting responsibilities; composition; nominations and appointments; terms of office; rules of order; record keeping; and communication mechanisms between the committee and other bodies (e.g., interdisciplinary care teams).

Organization Ethics

Committees should be aware of discussions about organization ethics. In 1995, the Joint Commission for Accreditation of Healthcare Organizations (JCAHO) added a section called "Organization Ethics" to its accreditation standards. It contains specific requirements for participating institutions to develop and institute policies addressing ethical issues related to daily business practices (e.g., billing, client transfers, marketing); contractual obligations with clients; and professional relationships within and beyond the organization. There also is a growing body of bioethics literature on this topic (Myser, Donehower, & Frank, 1999; Pentz, 1998, 1999; Potter, 1996, 1999; Renz & Eddy, 1996; Spencer, 1997; Spencer, Mills, Rorty, & Werhane, 2000; Werhane & Rorty, 2000).

Creation of an organization ethics program would involve an integration of the different perspectives brought to bear in cases of clinical (individual care) ethics, business ethics, and professional ethics. Various structures and mechanisms could result, including the creation of two ethics committees (clinical and organizational) or one committee with expanded responsibilities to deal with additional matters related to business and management issues. Movement in the direction of organization ethics is good because, as noted earlier, some issues that are presented as individual clinical issues would more properly be addressed at the organizational level. Therefore, although extended discussion of organization ethics is beyond the scope of this book, it would be worthwhile for committees to acquaint themselves with developments in this area and to keep track of issues that are, in essence, organizational (e.g., adequacy and/or distribution of resources; individual contractual issues).

WHO SHOULD BE REPRESENTED ON THE COMMITTEE?

An ethics committee should reflect the diversity of the community that it serves. A representative committee is composed of individuals with a wide range of backgrounds and has a balance between nursing home personnel and outside community members. A variety of backgrounds from which to choose might include: a trustee/board member; a resident; a resident's relative or surrogate; an outside community lay representative; resident advocate/ombudsman; president/facility administrator; nursing assistant; registered nurse; social worker; clergy/ pastoral care person; ethicist; physician; staff development director; lawyer/legal counsel. Maintaining a balance between persons who are employed by or closely affiliated with the nursing home and members drawn from other areas of the larger community has advantages. Nursing home personnel have insider knowledge of issues and concerns. They can facilitate communication between the committee and involved individuals. Outside community members may be able to take a more dispassionate view of situations. A committee that is balanced between in-house and outside members more easily maintains its credibility by its disassociation from the organizational hierarchy of the institution.

A committee might want to consider how its mix of backgrounds positions it to understand activities of resident care from a firsthand perspective. Resident, family, and nursing assistant representation may provide this. But power differentials and differences in life experiences and committee work among all members must be taken into account. For example, if the committee is overwhelmingly made up of upper echelon personnel or dominated by strong personalities, how comfortable are members to voice their opinions? What are the possibilities that their opinions will be guarded, overly accommodating, and predictable? These are questions that need to be asked and answered honestly and thoughtfully.

Consideration should be given to the personal qualities of potential committee members. Members who are thoughtful, reflective, critical thinkers, who accept and respect one another, have the patience to move slowly, and can tolerate ambiguity enhance the committee's effectiveness. Needed personal attributes are:

- **Humility**—A committee cannot function effectively without a fundamental commitment to the equality of all its members. Humility is expressed through willingness to work cooperatively with others, to listen well, and to respond respectfully. Members may disagree on certain points; but they need to debate issues in nonauthoritarian, nonadversarial ways. They should feel confident in sharing their true opinions and to rely on the good will of fellow members to hear without judgment, to accept without reprisals, and to treat committee member conversations in highest confidence.

- **Critical thinking skills**—Critical thinking requires a willingness to slow down and to think systematically about a situation, to have a questioning attitude, and to seek out additional information. Critical thinkers believe that there are at least two sides to every story. They want to find out all there is to know. They do not jump to conclusions and they realize that their own opinions might be wrong. Therefore, they want to hear from persons who have points of view that differ from their own. They can follow the logic of an argument or line of reasoning and are able to understand how different perspectives relate to the larger context of the situation.

  • **Patience**—Committee members need to exercise patience with themselves, with the situation, and with each other. Quick and obvious solutions need to be questioned. Reflection on issues requires a thoughtful attitude, willingness to imagine oneself in the place of another, and reluctance to move to answers until a full appreciation of concerns on all sides has been reached.

  • **Sense of humor**—Ethical dilemmas are not humorous and an ethics committee needs to take its work seriously. But individuals need not take themselves too seriously. The ability to laugh at one's own limitations gives others the courage to do the same. A healthy sense of humor also helps individuals find a saving grace, a brighter side, a touch of irony, or a sign of hope that opens up new insights and may free individuals to view a situation in another way. Appropriate use of humor can put people at ease and help equalize individuals, thus promoting the kind of comfortable atmosphere needed by the committee to generate good working relationships.

Basic Core Competencies

The American Society for Bioethics and Humanities (ASBH) report (1998) has identified some basic competencies (ethical assessment, process, and interpersonal skills) for health care ethics consultation. Although no single member need embody all of the skills, members' differing abilities, taken together, should meet the full range. And, in addition to individual competencies, the committee collectively should exhibit:

  • Skills necessary to identify the nature of the value uncertainty or conflict that underlies the need for ethics consultation.
  • Skills necessary to analyze the value uncertainty or conflict.
  • The ability to facilitate formal and informal meetings.
  • The ability to build moral consensus.
  • The ability to listen well and to communicate interest, respect, support, and empathy to involved parties.
  • The ability to elicit the moral views of involved parties.
  • The ability to represent the views of involved parties.

- The ability to enable the involved parties to communicate effectively and to be heard by other parties.
- The ability to recognize and attend to various relational barriers to communication. (ASBH, 1998, pp. 12, 15)

Developing competency is an ongoing process for individuals and groups. Attentiveness to core competencies will assist in selection and education of committee members. The process of preparing, attending, and participating in committee meetings is educational, also raising awareness and building members' confidence over time.

HOW BIG SHOULD THE COMMITTEE BE?

The size of ethics committees varies. There is no ideal number. A small size might be 8–10. A large committee might consist of 15–20 members. Advantages of larger committees are the ability to have more persons from outside the facility as members to enhance objectivity and the potential, if persons must be absent at times, for sufficient members to be left to carry on the work. The nature of the work will, in part, determine size. Member interest and reliability will be a truer test of effective size than abstract calculations. It may be useful to establish what will serve as a quorum at any meeting.

Leadership: The person who chairs needs to understand the committee's mission and functions and to have interpersonal skills that foster respect for all points of view and facilitate group process. In cooperation with the membership, chairs establish agendas, carry out the work of the group, and evaluate its progress. Having as chair an ethicist (or clergy, or physician, social worker, nurse, etc.) is not axiomatic. Requisite knowledge and leadership skills might be found in any member. The chair position also might be rotated.

HOW IS THE WORK OF THE COMMITTEE MANAGED?

Members of a newly established group can become acquainted with each other through reading and discussing educational materials that orient them to conversation and debate about ethical issues. Published examples of ethical cases or those in this book might serve as a basis for practice discussions. Practical matters of time, place, and frequency of meetings also will need to be discussed.

Constitutional and organizational issues. The committee needs to develop its own written guidelines about the following:

- Constitution—organizational placement and reporting responsibilities.
- Charge—committee purpose and functions.
  For example, to address ethical issues—not to make decisions, but to gather facts and provide informed advice; to assist in formulation of policies; to educate itself, staff, and others; to provide individual case reviews.
- Composition—representation, including ex-officio and appointed positions.
- Process for nominations, appointments, and removal of members.
- Terms of office for members who do not serve ex-officio—including conditions of reappointment and arrangements for balancing change and continuity in committee membership and establishment of a quorum.
- Case review process, format, and documentation (See sample record**).
- Function and format of minutes.
- Provisions for amending committee guidelines.

How Are Issues and Cases Brought Forward?

What written definition of an ethical issue/concern can the committee provide to guide the facility? For example: Ethical concerns arise when one or more interacting persons (e.g., residents, families, staff) feel discomfort about a resident life situation or decision. Discomfort often involves competing or conflicting values, which may be equally strong on each side (a dilemma). If open discussion results in consensus, the issue likely is one of communication. Ethical issues involve different perspectives about what should be done about something that may make reaching consensus through open discussion difficult.

Residents, their families, and nursing home staff come from diverse backgrounds. Thus, it is not unusual for their thoughts and actions to be guided by different personal values. Staff members not only may have different values from those of residents and families, but they also may have personal or professional values that differ from each other. For example, there may not be agreement among staff on *when* or *if* it is ever appropriate to tell residents who stay up all night that it is time to go to bed. There may be different value-based opinions between staff and families, among staff, among family members, and between residents, staff, and family members on such matters as how or when to follow advance directives, indications for the use of restraints, the advisability of intra-institutional transfers, and so on. Thus, there is no unitary "resident" or "family" or "staff" perspective on any given issue. Instead, there are many opportunities to examine the different ways in which people approach a resident-related concern and to determine together what values and priorities might most appropriately serve that person's best interests.

Who may bring an ethical issue/concern to the committee? Ethics consultation should be open to anyone. However, committees should try to pace themselves and not try to do everything at once. Ethical cases might arise from the multidisciplinary care conference process or various staff discussions. After the committee and staff members have gained a certain level of comfort and expertise in dialogue about common ethical issues, more consideration could be given to orientation of residents and families. The latter should not be encouraged to use the committee in place of appropriate channels of communication with staff. Residents and families also need to be oriented to available ombudsman (advocacy) services, which offer another avenue for investigating complaints and working with professional staff to resolve quality of life and care concerns. Ombudsmen are valuable resources to nursing homes and ethics committees, usually trained in conflict resolution and sensitive to varied ways in which individuals respond to issues.

An advantage of starting out with cases forwarded by staff members is that in time they may become more oriented to the process and comfortable in working with the committee. It is common for staff to feel intimidated by an ethics case review because: (a) they may associate the process with wrongdoing and worry that they or someone else will be subject to blame; (b) they may be unclear about appropriate topics and feel pressured by lack of time; (c) they may feel insecure about suggesting cases or issues to bring forward for committee discussion; (d) they may feel uncomfortable and self-conscious about their ability to present and discuss issues in committee; (e) they may fear retaliation from others for raising particular concerns; or (f) they may have a concrete black-and-white view of situations that does not recognize the potential in a diversity of opinions and perspectives that might be beneficial in seeking more insightful solutions. Overcoming indecision and hesitancy on the part of individuals involves building trust and confidence. Committees need to consider what the nursing home's ethical climate is like. A comfortable ethical climate is one in which staff feel appreciated and respected; where their opinions are sought out and listened to; and where their concerns are addressed in caring and nonjudgmental ways. It also is one in which the organizational mission is consistent with and visible in everyday practice. And it is one in which values embodied in its mission, policies, and code of ethics are shared by personnel at every organizational level (Spencer et al., 2000).

Another barrier to staff participation is scheduling. Committees should consider what meeting times conflict the least with staff work schedules. However, administrators and supervisors also should be encouraged to enable staff to participate. They should particularly ensure that those who have the best knowledge of and closest relationships with the resident's situation (e.g., nursing assistants, housekeepers) are able to attend.

Finally, staff interest in ongoing participation will depend on the committee's practical impact on their lives. If they perceive that committee members are able to grasp the realities that they face and contribute ideas that are useful and supportive in their work, a partnership will have been forged. And through the interest and commitment of staff, the most helpful ways to involve residents and families will be found.

How shall the issue/concern be presented to the committee? Members should receive in advance a case narrative that describes the resident situation, summarizes diverse views held by individuals, and lists questions for committee consideration. Helpful resource material (e.g., a relevant article and/or policy) also may be included. Proper names and identifiers should be omitted to maintain confidentiality. But removing names and identifiers does not of itself ensure confidentiality. Some committee members cannot help knowing individuals' identities. Therefore, members must understand that all committee business is confidential in nature. (The issue of confidentiality is discussed further below.)

WHAT PROCESSES AND PROCEDURES ARE FOLLOWED?

Documentation. Administrative review and advice of legal counsel should be sought on all matters involving record keeping and documentation. Committees should be informed about the issue of discoverability (laws that apply to committee records and reports related to committee activities) and indemnification protection. Members who are qualified to give advice in legal matters are critical committee assets. But assurance of documented support from administrative/governing nursing home bodies covering all committee activities is equally important. Ethics committee records might be expected to follow a consistent format and be kept in a separate confidential file (see sample record**).

Accountability. Someone on the committee needs to have had direct contact with the involved individuals (residents, families, and staff) to ensure that their perspectives, values, and preferences are represented adequately. Decisions about who to invite to meet with the committee should be made on a case-by-case basis, but all parties should be informed about the case review and resulting recommendations. Reporting mechanisms need to be established to communicate recommendations to interested parties not involved in committee discussion, for example, through the interdisciplinary care team. The committee also needs to have a way to receive feedback on outcomes of actions related to its recommendations and any remaining concerns. Members should consider whether or not issues raised by cases should be further pursued in the form of educational sessions or new/revised policies.

Confidentiality. Actions that the committee will take to respect the privacy of residents and other involved persons should be described in writing. Individuals' *moral right to privacy* involves all means used to keep personal information private. Because residents and their families lose some control over privacy when care must be coordinated by a number of other people, they must be assured of confidentiality. All committee members must understand and be regularly reminded that discussion of cases outside of committee, except through established communication channels with those directly involved in the resident's care and treatment, is a breach of confidentiality.

In addition to their moral rights, individuals have a *legal right to privacy*. Therefore, the committee needs to obtain and follow the advice of legal counsel to be sure that all of its policies and procedures take residents' rights under the law into account. For example, advice should be sought from legal counsel and nursing home administration on the format and amount of detail to include in committee records and communications as well the form and nature of information that should be recorded regarding ethics consultations in a resident's medical record.

Cases brought to ethics committees may be seen as valuable teaching tools for care professionals within and outside of the nursing home. Traditionally, presenters of clinical cases at teaching institutions or professional meetings and conferences observe persons' rights to confidentiality by being careful not to disclose names or other information that could reveal an individual's identity. This may include altering various aspects of the case to further reduce the possibility of linking the issues under discussion to a known person. Ensuring confidentiality is of special concern with vulnerable populations—for example, children and all institutionalized persons, especially adults lacking competency to give consent. Therefore, the committee's first and most important duty is to serve the best interests of the resident. And it must be careful to observe persons' rights to confidentiality in exercising educational duties for professional service through discussion of case-related issues. Usually, the many similarities that arise across multiple cases make it possible to focus on generic issues and types of situations in ways that maintain privacy and do not rely exclusively on the details of a particular case.

NOW WHAT?

Established committees sometimes experience needs to redirect, or reenergize themselves. Although solutions will vary, possible approaches may include:

Taking stock. Members could examine past cases and discuss common themes and patterns. Discussion outcomes might involve ideas for educational activities, review of policies and procedures, or an inventory and update of available resource material (see sample resources). A formal review of the committee's history and progress also can be validating and/or it may identify new needs (e.g., membership turnover requiring re-orientation efforts).

Trying something new. A committee could sponsor community meetings where anyone within the facility (residents, families, staff) is welcomed to share perspectives on common issues. It also could write a feature article or invite readers' questions about issues through established community newsletters. Or, rather than waiting for referred cases, it might randomly or purposefully select cases according to some criterion (e.g., the most newly admitted or the longest stay resident) for an overall review of quality of life/quality of care (Powers, 2000). This proactive approach is based on the assumption that ethical concerns are inherent in and unique to every individual's situation.

Recommitting. Reviewing the committee's mission and guidelines can become a means of recommitting to the spirit of the group when it was originally formed. This also could involve a social ritual (e.g., celebration, member recognition), a retreat, or a benefit (e.g., funding for attendance at a workshop or conference, a meal or refreshments at meetings). Knowledge of the membership and imagination should suggest tangible and symbolic ways to rekindle enthusiasm and reward individuals' efforts.

Sample Case Review Record**

Ethics Committee Case Number:
Medical Record Number:
Date of Review:
Individuals Present:

Ethical Issues: *Limits of Intervention—Negative moral rights*
Mr. Q was admitted from the hospital with a dysfunctional gastric feeding tube that must either be removed or replaced. His advance directive specifically states "no nasal or gastric feeding tube" but, although distressed that he is dying and that the presence of the feeding tube is contrary to his stated wishes, family members feel guilty about agreeing that tube feeding should be discontinued. They want to abide by Mr. Q's current wishes as determined by a physician. Some staff members are distressed because they believe that Mr. Q's nonverbal behavior suggests that he does not want the feeding tube. Others share the family's discomfort in withdrawing nutritional support, though not their hope for a rational response from Mr. Q.
Competing goods (values) are: *It is good to respect Mr. Q's previously stated wishes vs. it is good to provide fluids and nourishment.* Institutional policy: *Advance directives are part of interinstitutional transfer, which is affirmed to be a good policy.* Resident actions: *Pushes caregivers' hands away when they attempt tube-related care.* Dementia: *Diagnosed late-stage with lethargy and absence of lucid conversation.* Related sources: *McCann et al, 1994: Comfort care for terminally ill patients: The appropriate use of nutrition and hydration; Fordyce, 2000: Dehydration near the end of life.*

Resident Preferences: *Mr. Q was of sound mind when he wrote his advance directive with the help of his family and attending physician. He requested the absence of heroic measures and specifically stated that he did not want a nasal or gastric feeding tube in the event that he was unable to take oral nutrition. The physician's determination is that, currently, Mr. Q lacks capacity to express his wishes regarding artificial feeding. Family members, as his surrogates, are not comfortable in sanctioning this stipulation.*

Quality of Life: *Mr. Q cannot take food and fluids orally and is actively dying. He has intermittent vomiting and discomfort associated with the dysfunctional feeding tube. Surgical correction of the malfunction would require rehospitalization.*

Contextual Features: *Family members need emotional support and information about withdrawal of food and fluids and palliative (comfort) care measures.*

Recommendation: Support removal of the feeding tube, based on the resident's advance directive.

Sample Resources

BOOKS (See references for full citations.)

Bayley. (1999). *Elegy for Iris.*
R. A. Kane, & Caplan. (1990). *Everyday ethics: Resolving dilemmas in nursing home life.*
Kovach. (1997). *Late-stage dementia care: A basic guide.*
Mace, & Rabins. (1990). *The 36-hour day: A family guide to caring for persons with Alzheimer disease, related dementing illnesses, and memory loss in later life.*
Rabins, Lyketsos, & Steele. (1999). *Practical dementia care.*
Shenk. (2001). *Alzheimer's: Portrait of an epidemic.*
Snowdon. (2001). *Aging with grace: What the nun study teaches us about leading longer, healthier, and more meaningful lives.*

JOURNALS

ALZHEIMER'S DISEASE AND GERONTOLOGY-RELATED TOPICS

Alzheimer's Care Quarterly; Alzheimer Disease & Associated Disorders; American Journal of Alzheimer's Disease and Other Dementias; American Journal of Hospice & Palliative Care; Annals of Long-Term Care; Generations; Geriatrics; Geriatric Nursing; Journal of Aging Studies; International Journal of Aging and Human Development; Journal of the American Geriatrics Society; Journal of Cross-Cultural Gerontology; Journal of Gerontological Nursing; The Gerontologist; The Journals of Gerontology

ETHICS

Bioethics Forum; Cambridge Quarterly of Healthcare Ethics; Hastings Center Report; HEC [HealthCare Ethics Committee] Forum; Kennedy

Institute of Ethics Journal; Law, Medicine, and Ethics; The Journal of
Clinical Ethics

WEB SITES

Alzheimer's Disease and Related Disorders Association
  www.alz.org
Alzheimer's Disease Education and Referral Center
  www.alzheimers.org
American Association of Homes and Services for the Aging
  www.aahsa.org
American Society for Bioethics and Humanities (ASBH)
  www.asbh.org
American Nurses Association Center for Ethics and Human Rights
  www.nursingworld.org/ethics
Kennedy Institute of Ethics/Georgetown University
  www.georgetown.edu/research/kie

References

Agency for Health Care Policy and Research (1996a). *Early Alzheimer's disease: A guide for patients and families.* Silver Spring, MD: Author.

Agency for Health Care Policy and Research (1996b). *Recognition and initial assessment of Alzheimer's disease and related dementias: Clinical practice guideline and Quick reference guide for clinicians.* Silver Spring, MD: Author.

Albert, S. M., & Logsdon, R. G. (Eds.). (2000). *Assessing quality of life in Alzheimer's disease.* New York: Springer.

Alzheimer's Disease and Related Disorders Association. (2001a). General statistics and demographics. Retrieved 6-28-02 from www.alz.org.

Alzheimer's Disease and Related Disorders Association. (2001b). Policy statement on driving and dementia. Chicago: Author.

Alzheimer's Disease and Related Disorders Association. (2002). Alzheimer's Association Safe Return Fact Sheet. Chicago: Author.

American Geriatrics Society, British Geriatric Society, & American Academy of Orthopaedic Surgeons Panel on Falls Prevention. (2001). Guideline for the prevention of falls in older persons. *Annals of Long-Term Care, 9*(11), 42–54, 57.

American Psychiatric Association. (1994). *Diagnostic and statistical manual (4th ed.).* Washington, DC: Author.

American Society for Bioethics and Humanities. (1998). *Core competencies for health care ethics consultation.* Glenville, IL: Author.

Baer, W. M., & Hanson, L. C. (2000). Families' perception of the added value of hospice in the nursing home. *Journal of the American Geriatrics Society, 48,* 879–882.

Barba, B. E., Tesh, A. S., & Courts, N. F. (2002). Promoting thriving in nursing homes: The Eden Alternative. *Journal of Gerontological Nursing, 28*(3), 7–13.

Barkan, B. (1995). The regenerative community: The Live Oak Living Center and the quest for autonomy, self-esteem, and connection in elder care. In L. M. Gamroth, J. Semradek, & E. M. Tornquist (Eds.), *Enhancing autonomy in long-term care: Concepts and strategies* (pp. 169–192). New York: Springer.

Bayley, J. (1999). *Elegy for Iris.* New York: St. Martin's Press.

Beauchamp, T., & Childress, J. (1983). *Principles of biomedical ethics.* New York: Oxford University Press.

Beck, C., Heacock, P., Rapp, C. G., & Mercer, S. O. (1993). Assisting cognitively impaired elders with activities of daily living. *American Journal of Alzheimer's Care and Related Disorders & Research, 8*(6), 11–20.

Bellah, R. N. (1982). Social science as practical reason. *The Hastings Center Report, 12*(5), 32–39.

Berger, J. T. (2000). Sexuality and intimacy in the nursing home: A romantic couple of mixed cognitive capacities. *The Journal of Clinical Ethics, 11,* 309–313.

Boyd, C. (1994). Residents first: A long-term care facility introduces a social model that puts residents in control. *Health Progress, 75*(7), 34–39, 50.

Boyd, K. M., Higgs, R., & Pinching, A. J. (1997). *The new dictionary of medical ethics.* London: BMJ Publishing Group.

Buckwalter, K. C. (2002). Special Issue: End-of-Life Research: Focus on Older Populations (Guest Editor). *The Gerontologist, 42,* Special Issue III.

Buettner, L. L. (1998). A team approach to dynamic programming on the special care unit. *Journal of Gerontological Nursing, 24*(1), 23–30.

Butler, R. (1968). *Why survive? Being old in America.* New York: Harper & Row.

Callahan, D. (1984). Autonomy: A moral good, not a moral obsession. *The Hastings Center Report, 14*(5), 40–42.

Capezuti, E., Strumpf, N. E., Evans, L. K., Grisso, J. A., & Maislin, G. (1998). The relationship between physical restraint removal and falls and injuries among nursing home residents. *Journals of Gerontology: Series A, Biological & Medical Sciences, 53*(1), M47–M52.

Cassel, C. K., & Foley, K. M. (1999). *Principles for the care of patients at the end of life: An emerging consensus among the specialties of medicine.* New York: Millbank Memorial Fund.

Castle, N. G., Fogel, B., & Mor, V. (1997). Risk factors for physical restraint use in nursing homes: Pre- and post-implementation of the Nursing Home Reform Act. *The Gerontologist, 37,* 737–747.

Castle, N. G., & Fogel, B. (1998). Characteristics of nursing homes that are restraint-free. *The Gerontologist, 38,* 181–188.

Chitsey, A. M., Haight, B. K., & Jones, M. M. (2002). Snoezelen: A multisensory environmental intervention. *Journal of Gerontological Nursing, 28*(3), 41–49.

Cohen-Mansfield, J., Rabinovich, B. A., Lipson, S., Fein, A., Gerber, B., Weisman, S., et al. (1991). The decision to execute a durable power of attorney for health care and preferences regarding the utilization of life-sustaining treatments in nursing home residents. *Archives of Internal Medicine, 151,* 289–294.

Coleman, C., & Petruzzelli, M. (2001). Decision making for residents without surrogates. In M. D. Mezey & N. N. Dubler, *Voices of decisions in nursing homes* (pp. 65–72). New York: United Hospital Fund.

Coleman, M. T., Looney, S., O'Brien, J., Ziegler, C., Pastorino, C. A., & Turner, C. (2002). The Eden Alternative: Findings after 1 year of implementation. *Journals of Gerontology: Series A, Biological & Medical Sciences, 57*(7), M422–M427.

Collopy, B. J. (1992). The use of restraints in long-term care: The ethical issues. *American Association of Homes for the Aging White Paper.* Washington, DC: American Association of Homes for the Aging.

Cullum, C. M., & Rosenberg, R. N. (1998). Memory loss—When is it Alzheimer disease? *JAMA, 279,* 1689–1690.

Curry, L., Porter, M., Michalski, M., & Gruman, C. (2000). Individualized care: Perceptions of certified nurse's aides. *Journal of Gerontological Nursing, 26*(7), 45–51.

Danis, M., & Churchill, L. R. (1991). Autonomy and the common weal. *The Hastings Center Report, 21*(1), 25–31.

Davis, D. S. (1991). Rich cases: The ethics of thick description. *The Hastings Center Report, 21*(4), 12–16.

Detweiler, M. B., Trinkle, D. B., & Anderson, M. S. (2002). Wander gardens: Expanding the dementia treatment environment. *Annals of Long-Term Care, 10*(3), 68–74.

Drought, T. S., & Koenig, B. A. (2002). "Choice" in end-of-life decision making: Researching fact or fiction? *The Gerontologist, 42*, Special Issue III, 114–128.

Dubler, N., & Nimmons, D. (1992). *Ethics on call: Taking charge of life-and-death choices in today's health care system.* New York: Vintage Books.

Dunbar, J. M., Neufeld, R. R., White, H. C., & Libow, L. S. (1996). Retrain, don't restrain: The educational intervention of the National Nursing Home Restraint Removal Project. *The Gerontologist, 36*, 539–542.

Durnbaugh, T., Haley, B., & Roberts, S. (1996). Assessing problem feeding behaviors in midstage Alzheimer's disease. *Geriatric Nursing, 17*(2), 63–67.

Emson, H. E. (1995). Rights, duties, and limits of autonomy. *Cambridge Quarterly Healthcare Ethics, 4*(1), 7–11.

Epps, C. D. (2001). Recognizing pain in the institutionalized elder with dementia. *Geriatric Nursing, 22*(2), 71–77.

Ersek, M., Kraybill, B. M., & Hansberry, J. (2000). Assessing the educational needs and concerns of nursing home staff regarding end-of-life care. *Journal of Gerontological Nursing, 26*(10), 16–26.

Evans, D. A., Scherr, P. A., Cook, N. R., Albert, M. S., Funkenstein, H. H., Beckett, L. A., et al. (1992). The impact of Alzheimer's disease in the United States population. In R. M. Suzman, D. P. Willis, & K. G. Manton (Eds.), *The oldest old* (pp. 283–299). New York: Oxford University Press.

Evans, J. H. (2000). A sociological account of the growth of principlism. *The Hastings Center Report, 30*(5), 31–38.

Evans, L. K., & Strumpf, N. E. (1989). Tying down the elderly: A review of the literature on physical restraint. *Journal of the American Geriatrics Society, 37*, 65–74.

Evans, L. K., Strumpf, N. E., Allen-Taylor, S. L., Capezuti, E., Maislin, G., & Jacobsen, B. (1997). A clinical trial to reduce restraints in nursing homes. *Journal of the American Geriatrics Society, 45*, 675–681.

Finucane, T. E., Christmas, C., & Travis, K. (1999). Tube feeding in patients with advanced dementia: A review of the evidence. *JAMA, 282*, 1365–1370.

Foner, N. (1994a). *The caregiving dilemma: Work in an American nursing home.* Berkeley, CA: University of California Press.

Foner, N. (1994b). Nursing home aides: Saints or monsters? *The Gerontologist, 34*, 245–250.

Foner. (1995). The hidden injuries of bureaucracy: Work in an American nursing home. *Human Organization, 54*, 229–237.

Fordyce, M. (2000). Dehydration near the end of life. *Annals of Long-Term Care, 8*(5), 29–33.

Fowler, M. D. M., & Levine-Ariff, J. (1987). *Ethics at the bedside.* Philadelphia: JB Lippincott.

Gates, D. M., Fitzwater, E., & Meyer, U. (1999). Violence against caregivers in nursing homes. *Journal of Gerontological Nursing, 25*(4), 12–22.

Goffman, I. (1961). *Asylums: Essays on the social situation of mental patients and other inmates.* Garden City, NY: Doubleday.

Gubrium, J. F. (1975). *Living and dying at Murray Manor.* New York: St. Martin's Press.

Gubrium, J. F. (1993). *Speaking of life: Horizons of meaning for nursing home residents.* Chicago: Aldine de Gruyter.

Gubrium, J. F. (1995). Perspective and story in nursing home ethnography. In J. N. Henderson & M. D. Vesperi (Eds.), *The culture of long term care: Nursing home ethnography* (pp. 23–36). Westport, CT: Bergin & Garvey.

Happ, M. B., Williams, C. C., Strumpf, N. E., & Burger, S. G. (1996). Individualized care for frail elders: Theory and practice. *Journal of Gerontological Nursing, 22*(3), 6–14.

Harrington, C., Kovner, C., Mezey, M., Kayser-Jones, J., Burger, S., Mohler, M., et al. (2000). Experts recommend minimum nurse staffing standards for nursing facilities in the United States. *The Gerontologist, 40,* 5–16.

Harris, D. K., & Benson, M. L. (2000). Theft in nursing homes. *Journal of Gerontological Nursing, 26*(8), 33–34.

Hebrew Home for the Aged at Riverdale, New York. (2002a). Resident sexuality in the nursing home (staff education manual). Author. (Distributor: Terra Nova Films.)

Hebrew Home for the Aged at Riverdale, New York. (2002b). Freedom of sexual expression: Dementia and resident rights in long-term care facilities (video). Author. (Distributor: Terra Nova Films.)

Henderson, J. N. (1981). Nursing home housekeepers: Indigenous agents of psychosocial support. *Human Organization, 40,* 300–305.

Henderson, J. N. (1987). When a professor turns nurse aide. *Provider, 13,* 8–12.

Henderson. (1995). The culture of care in a nursing home: Effects of a medicalized model of long-term care. In J. N. Henderson & M. D. Vesperi (Eds.), *The culture of long-term care: Nursing home ethnography* (pp. 37–54). Westport, CT: Bergin & Garvey.

Henderson, J. N., & Vesperi, M. D. (Eds.). (1995). *The culture of long term care: Nursing home ethnography.* Westport, CT: Bergin & Garvey.

Henkel, G. (2000). More to the "Eden Alternative" than meets the eye. *Caring for the Ages, 1*(4), 21–23.

Hoeffer, B., Rader, J., McKenzie, D., Lavelle, M., & Stewart, B. (1997). Reducing aggressive behavior during bathing cognitively impaired nursing home residents. *Journal of Gerontological Nursing, 23*(5), 16–23.

Hofland, B. F. (2001). Ethics and aging: A historical perspective. In M. B. Holstein & P. B. Mitzen (Eds.), *Ethics in community-based elder care* (pp. 19–30). New York: Springer.

Horgas, A. L., & Tsai, P.-F. (1998). Analgesic drug prescription and use in cognitively impaired nursing home residents. *Nursing Research, 47,* 235–242.

Howe, E. G. (2000). Improving treatment for patients who are elderly and have dementia. *The Journal of Clinical Ethics, 11,* 291–303.

Hurley, A. C., Volicer, L., Rempusheski, V. F., & Fry, S. T. (1995). Reaching consensus: The process of recommending treatment decisions for Alzheimer's patients. *Advances in Nursing Science, 18*(2), 33–43.

Janzen, W. (2001). Long-term care for older adults: The role of the family. *Journal of Gerontological Nursing, 27*(2), 36–43.

Jennings, B. (2000). A life greater than the sum of its sensations: Ethics, dementia, and the quality of life. In S. M. Albert & R. G. Logsdon (Eds.), *Assessing quality of life in Alzheimer's disease* (pp. 165–178). New York: Springer.

Jirovec, M. M., & Wells, T. J. (1990). Urinary incontinence in nursing home residents with dementia: The mobility-cognition paradigm. *Applied Nursing Research, 3,* 112–117.

Jones, M. M., & Haight, B. K. (2002). Environmental transformations: An integrative review. *Journal of Gerontological Nursing, 28*(3), 23–27.

Jonsen, A. R., Siegler, M., & Winslade, W. J. (1998). *Clinical ethics: A practical approach to ethical decisions in clinical medicine* (4th ed.). New York: McGraw-Hill.

Jonsen, A. R., & Toulmin, S. (1988). *The abuse of casuistry: A history of moral reasoning.* Berkeley, CA: University of California Press.

Kamel, H. K. (2001). Sexuality in aging: Focus on institutionalized elderly. *Annals of Long-Term Care, 9*(5), 64–72.

Kane, R. A., & Caplan, A. L. (1990). *Everyday ethics: Resolving dilemmas in nursing home life.* New York: Springer.

Kane, R. A., Kane, R. L., & Ladd, R. C. (1998). *The heart of long-term care.* New York: Oxford University Press.

Kane, R. A., & Levin, C. A. (2001). Who's safe? Who's sorry?: The duty to protect the safety of the HCBS consumers. In M. B. Holstein & P. B. Mitzen (Eds.), *Ethics in community-based elder care* (pp. 217–233). New York: Springer.

Kane, R. L., Williams, C. C., Williams, T. F., & Kane, R. A. (1993). Restraining restraints: Changes in a standard of care. In G. S. Omenn, J. E. Fielding, & L. B. Lave (Eds.), *Annual Review of Public Health, 14,* 545–584.

Kayser-Jones, J. S. (1981). *Old, alone, and neglected: Care of the aged in the United States and Scotland.* Berkeley, CA: University of California Press.

Kayser-Jones, J. S. (1991). The impact of the environment on the quality of care in nursing homes: A social-psychological perspective. *Holistic Nursing Practice, 5*(3), 29–38.

Kayser-Jones, J. S. (1992). Culture, environment, and restraints: A conceptual model for research and practice. *Journal of Gerontological Nursing, 18*(11), 13–20.

Kayser-Jones, J. S. (1996). Mealtime in nursing homes: The importance of individualized care. *Journal of Gerontological Nursing, 22*(3), 26–31.

Kayser-Jones, J. S. (1997). Inadequate staffing at mealtime: Implications for nursing and health policy. *Journal of Gerontological Nursing, 23*(8), 14–21.

Kayser-Jones, J. S. (2000). A case study of the death of an older woman in a nursing home: Are nursing care practices in compliance with ethical guidelines? *Journal of Gerontological Nursing, 26*(9), 48–54.

Kayser-Jones, J. S. (2002). The experience of dying: An ethnographic nursing home study. *The Gerontologist, 42,* Special Issue III, 11–19.

Kayser-Jones, J. S., Davis, A., Wiener, C. L., & Higgens, S. S. (1989). An ethical analysis of an elder's treatment. *Nursing Outlook, 37,* 267–270.

Kayser-Jones, J. S., & Pengilly, K. (1999). Dysphagia among nursing home residents. *Geriatric Nursing, 20*(2), 77–82.

Kayser-Jones, J. S., & Schell, E. (1997a). The effect of staffing on the quality of care at mealtime. *Nursing Outlook, 45,* 64–72.

Kayser-Jones, J. S., & Schell, E. (1997b). The mealtime experience of a cognitively impaired elder: Ineffective and effective strategies. *Journal of Gerontological Nursing, 23*(7), 33–39.

Kelley, L. S., Swanson, E., Maas, M. L., & Tripp-Reimer, T. (1999). Family visitation on special care units. *Journal of Gerontological Nursing, 25*(2), 14–21.

Kitwood, T. (1998). Toward a theory of dementia care: Ethics and interaction. *The Journal of Clinical Ethics, 9*(1), 23–34.

Kovach, C. R. (1997). *Late-stage dementia care: A basic guide.* Bristol, PA: Taylor & Francis.

Kovach, C. R. (1998). Nursing home dementia care units: Providing a continuum of care rather than aging in place. *Journal of Gerontological Nursing, 24*(4), 30–36.

Kraker, K., & Vajdik, C. (1997). Designing the environment to make bathing pleasant in nursing homes. *Journal of Gerontological Nursing, 23*(5), 50–51.

Leake, C. D. (1975). *Percival's medical ethics.* Huntington, NY: R. E. Kreiger.

Lustbader, W. (2001). The pioneer challenge: A radical change in the culture of nursing homes. In L. S. Noelker & Z. Harel (Eds.), *Linking quality of long-term care and quality of life* (pp. 185–203). New York: Springer.

Lynn, J. (1997). Measuring quality of care at the end of life: A statement of principles. *Journal of the American Geriatrics Society, 45,* 526–527.

Maas, M. L., Specht, J. P., Weiler, K., Buckwalter, K. C., & Turner, B. (1998). Special care units for people with Alzheimer's disease: Only for the privileged few? *Journal of Gerontological Nursing, 24*(3), 28–37.

Mace, N. L., & Rabins, P. V. (1999). *The 36-hour day: A family guide to caring for persons With Alzheimer disease, related dementing illnesses, and memory loss in later life* (3rd ed.). Baltimore: The Johns Hopkins University Press.

Mahoney, E. K., Volicer, L., & Hurley, A. C. (2000). *Management of challenging behaviors in dementia.* Baltimore: Health Professions Press.

Mason, L. D. (1995). Ethnography and the nursing home ombudsman. In J. N. Henderson & M. D. Vesperi (Eds.), *The culture of long term care: Nursing home ethnography* (pp. 71–91). Westport, CT: Bergin & Garvey.

McCann, R. (1999). Lack of evidence about tube feeding—Food for thought. *JAMA, 282,* 1380–1381.

McCann, R. M., Hall, W. J., & Groth-Juncker (1994). Comfort care for terminally ill patients: The appropriate use of nutrition and hydration. *JAMA, 272,* 1263–1266.

McCrae, C. S., & Lichstein, K. L. (2002). Managing insomnia in long-term care. *Annals of Long-Term Care, 10*(4), 38–43.

Mezey, M. D., Dubler, N. N., Bottrell, M., Mitty, E., Ramsey, G., Post, L. F., et al. (2001). Guidelines for end-of-life care in nursing homes: Principles and recommendations. New York: New York University Division of Nursing, the John A. Hartford institute for Geriatric Nursing and the Montefiore Medical Center Division of Bioethics.

Mezey, M., Dubler, N. N., Mitty, E., & Brody, A. A. (2002). What impact do setting and transitions have on the quality of life at the end of life and the quality of the dying process? *The Gerontologist, 42,* Special Issue III, 54–67.

Mezey, M., Miller, L. L., & Linton-Nelson, L. (1999). Caring for caregivers of frail elders at the end of life. *Generations, 23,* 44–51.

Mezey, M., Teresi, J., Ramsey, G.,, Mitty, E., & Bobrowitz, T. (2000). Decision-making capacity to execute a health care proxy: Development and testing of guidelines. *Journal of the American Geriatrics Society, 48,* 179–187.

Miles, S., & Irving, P. (1992). Deaths caused by physical restraints. *The Gerontologist, 32,* 762–766.

Miles, S. H., & Parker, K. (1999). Sexuality in the nursing home: Iatrogenic loneliness. *Generations, 23*(1), 36–43.

Miller, L. L., Nelson, L. L., & Mezey, M. (2000). Comfort and pain relief in dementia: Awakening a new beneficence. *Journal of Gerontological Nursing, 26*(9), 32–40.

Miller, M. F. (1997). Physically aggressive resident behavior during hygienic care. *Journal of Gerontological Nursing, 23*(5), 24–39.

Moss, F. E., & Halamandaris, V. J. (1977). *Too old, too sick, too bad: Nursing homes in America.* Germantown, MD: Aspen Systems Corp.

Moss, R. J., & La Puma, J. (1991). The ethics of mechanical restraints. *Hastings Center Report, 21*(1), 22–25.

Myser, C., Donehower, P., & Frank, C. (1999). Making the most of disequilibrium: Bridging the gap between clinical and organizational ethics in a newly merged healthcare organization. *The Journal of Clinical Ethics, 10,* 194–201.

National Institute of Neurological Disorders and Stroke. (2001). NINDS Pick's Disease Information Page. http://www.ninds.nih.gov/health-and-medical/disorders/picks_doc.htm

National Institute on Aging, National Institutes of Health. (1997). *Progress report on Alzheimer's disease.* Silver Spring, MD: Author.

O'Brien, H. L., Tetewsky, S. J., Avery, L. M., Cushman, L. A., Makous, W., & Duffy, C. J. (2001). Visual mechanisms of spatial disorientation in Alzheimer's disease. *Cerebral Cortex, 11,* 1083–1092.

O'Brien, M. (1989). *Anatomy of a nursing home: A new view of residential life.* Owings Mills, MD: National Health Publishing.

O'Rourke, D. J., Klaasen, K. S., & Sloan, J. A. (2001). Redesigning nighttime care for personal care residents. *Journal of Gerontological Nursing, 27*(7), 30–37.

Ouslander, J. G. (2000). Incontinence management in long-term care. *Annals of Long-Term Care, 8*(6), 35–41.

Peatfield, J. G., Futrell, M., & Cox, C. L. (2002). Wandering: An integrative review. *Journal of Gerontological Nursing, 28*(4), 44–50.

Pellegrino, E. D., & Thomasma, D. C. (1988). *For the patient's good: The restoration of beneficence in health care.* New York: Oxford University Press.

Pentz, R. D. (1998). Expanding into organizational ethics: The experience of one clinical ethics committee. *HEC Forum, 10,* 213–219.

Pentz, R. D. (1999). Beyond case consultation: An expanded model for organizational ethics. *The Journal of Clinical Ethics, 10,* 34–41.

Pillemer, K., Hegeman, C. R., Albright, B., & Henderson, C. (1998). Building bridges between families and nursing home staff: The Partners in Caregiving Program. *The Gerontologist, 38,* 499–503.

Post, S. G. (2000a). Commentary on "Sexuality and intimacy in the nursing home." *The Journal of Clinical Ethics, 11,* 314–317.

Post, S. G. (2000b). *The moral challenge of Alzheimer disease: Ethical issues from diagnosis to dying* (2nd ed.). Baltimore: The Johns Hopkins University Press.

Post, S. G. (2001). Tube feeding and advanced progressive dementia. *Hastings Center Report, 31*(1), 36–42.

Potter, R. L. (1996). From clinical ethics to organizational ethics: The second stage of the evolution of bioethics. *Bioethics Forum, 12,* 3–12.

Potter, R. L. (1999). On our way to integrated bioethics: Clinical/organizational/communal. *The Journal of Clinical Ethics, 10,* 171–177.

Powers, B. A. (1988a). Social networks, social support, and elderly institutionalized people. *Advances in Nursing Science, 10*(2), 40–58.

Powers, B. A. (1988b). Self-perceived health of elderly institutionalized people. *Journal of Cross-Cultural Gerontology, 3,* 299–321.

Powers, B. A. (1991). The meaning of nursing home friendships. *Advances in Nursing Science, 14*(2), 42–58.

Powers, B. A. (1992). The roles staff play in the social networks of elderly institutionalized people. *Social Science & Medicine, 34,* 1335–1343.

Powers, B. A. (1995). From the inside out: The world of the institutionalized elderly. In J. N. Henderson & M. D. Vesperi (Eds.), *The culture of long term care: Nursing home ethnography* (pp. 179–196). Westport, CT: Bergin & Garvey.

Powers, B. A. (1996). Relationships among older women living in a nursing home. *Journal of Women & Aging, 8*(3/4), 179–198.

Powers, B. A. (1997). Social support, social networks, and the problem of loneliness in elder care. In E. A. Swanson & T. Tripp-Reimer (Eds.), *Advances in gerontological nursing: Chronic illness and the older adult* (pp. 136–158). New York: Springer.

Powers, B. A. (2000). Everyday ethics of dementia care in nursing homes: A definition and taxonomy. *American Journal of Alzheimer's Disease, 15*(3), 143–151.

Powers, B. A. (2001). Ethnographic analysis of everyday ethics in the care of nursing home residents with dementia: A taxonomy. *Nursing Research, 50,* 332–339.

Powers, B. A. (In press). The significance of losing things for nursing home residents with dementia and their families. *Journal of Gerontological Nursing.*

Price, R. W. (1998). AIDS Dementia Complex: HIV Inside Knowledge Base Chapter. Center for HIV Information, University of California, San Francisco. http://hivinsite.ucsf.edu/Insite.jsp?doc=kb-04-01-03

Rabins, P. V., Lyketsos, C. G., & Steele, C. D. (1999). *Practical dementia care.* New York: Oxford University Press.

Rader, J. (1994). To bathe or not to bathe: That is the question. *Journal of Psychosocial Nursing, 32*(9), 53–54.

Rader, J. (1995). *Individualized dementia care: Creative, compassionate approaches.* New York: Springer.

Rader, J., Lavelle, M., Hoeffer, B., & McKenzie, D. (1996). Maintaining cleanliness: An individualized approach. *Journal of Gerontological Nursing, 22*(3), 32–38.

Reinhard, S. C., Barber, P. M., Mezey, M., Mitty, E. L., & Peed, J. A. (2002). Initiatives to promote the nursing workforce in geriatrics: A collaborative report. Available online at the following sites: The John A. Hartford Foundation http://www.hartfordign.org; Institute for the Future of Aging Services http://www.futureofaging.org; Rutgers >Center for State Health Policy http://www.cshp.rutgers.edu

Rempusheski, V. F., & Hurley, A. C. (2000). Advance directives and dementia. *Journal of Gerontological Nursing, 26*(9), 27–34.

Renz, D. O., & Eddy, W. B. (1996). Organizations, ethics, and health care: Building an ethics infrastructure for a new era. *Bioethics Forum, 12,* 13–20.

Richards, K. C., Sullivan, S. C., Phillips, R. L., Beck, C. K., & Overton-McCoy, A. L. (2001). The effect of individualized activities on the sleep of nursing home residents who are cognitively impaired: A pilot study. *The Journal of Gerontological Nursing, 27*(9), 30–37.

Rubenstein, L. (2000). Approaching falls in older persons. *Annals of Long-Term Care, 8*(8), 61–64.

Ryan, A. A., & Scullion, H. F. (2000). Family and staff perceptions of the role of families in nursing homes. *Journal of Advanced Nursing, 32,* 626–634.

Sabat, S. R. (1998). Voices of Alzheimer's disease sufferers: A call for treatment based on personhood. *The Journal of Clinical Ethics, 9,* 35–48.

Sandelowski, M. (1996). One is the liveliest number: The case orientation of qualitative research. *Research in Nursing & Health, 19,* 525–529.

Savishinsky, J. S. (1991). *The ends of time: Life and work in a nursing home.* Westport, CT: Bergin & Garvey.

Savishinsky, J. S. (1995). In and out of bounds: The ethics of respect in studying nursing homes. In J. N. Henderson & M. D. Vesperi (Eds.), *The culture of long term care: Nursing home ethnography* (pp. 93–109). Westport, CT: Bergin & Garvey.

Scarpinato, N., Schell, E., & Kagan, S. H. (2000). Nursing rounds from the University of Pennsylvania: Kitty's dilemma. *American Journal of Nursing, 100*(3), 49–51.

Schnelle, J. F., Alessi, C. A., Al-Samarrai, N. R., Fricker, R. D., & Ouslander, J. G. (1999). The nursing home at night: Effects of an intervention on noise, light, and sleep. *Journal of the American Geriatrics Society, 47,* 430–438.

Sellers, C. R., & Angerame, M. C. (2002). HIV/AIDS in older adults: A case study and discussion. *AACN Clinical Issues, 13,* 5–21.

Shenk, D. (2001). *Alzheimer's: Portrait of an epidemic.* New York: Doubleday.

Shield, R. R. (1988). *Uneasy endings: Daily life in an American nursing home.* Ithaca, NY: Cornell University Press.

Shield, R. R. (1995). Ethics in the nursing home: Cases, choices, and issues. In J. N. Henderson & M. D. Vesperi (Eds.), *The culture of long term care: Nursing home ethnography* (pp. 111–126). Westport, CT: Bergin & Garvey.

Sloane, P. D., Zimmerman, S., Suchindran, C., Reed, P., Wang, L., Boustani, M., et al. (2002). The public health impact of Alzheimer's disease, 2000–2050: Potential implication of treatment advances. In J. E. Fielding, R. C. Brownson, & B. Starfield (Eds.), *Annual Review of Public Health, 23,* 213–231.

Sloane, P. O., Matthew, L. J., Scarborough, M., Desai, J. R., Koch, G. G., & Tangen, C. (1991). Physical and pharmacologic restraint of nursing home residents with dementia: Impact of specialized units. *JAMA, 265,* 1278–1282.

Small, G. W., Rabins, P. V., Barry, P. P., Buckholtz, N. S., DeKosky, S. T., Ferris, S. H., et al. (1997). Diagnosis and treatment of Alzheimer disease and related disorders: Consensus statement of the American Association for Geriatric Psychiatry, the Alzheimer's Association, and the American Geriatrics Society. *JAMA, 278,* 1363–1371.

Snowdon, D. (2001). *Aging with grace: What the nun study teaches us about leading longer, healthier, and more meaningful lives.* New York: Bantam Books.

Spencer, E. M. (1997). A new role for institutional ethics committees: Organizational ethics. *The Journal of Clinical Ethics, 8,* 372–376.

Spencer, E. M., Mills, A. E., Rorty, M. V., & Werhane, P. H. (2000). *Organizational ethics in health care.* New York: Oxford University Press.

Stafford, P. B. (1995). Foreword. In J. N. Henderson & M. D. Vesperi (Eds.), *The culture of long term care: Nursing home ethnography* (pp. ix–x). Westport, CT: Bergin & Garvey.

Strumpf, N., Robinson, J. P., Wagner, J. S., & Evans, L. (1998). *Restraint-free care: Individualized approaches for frail elders.* New York: Springer.

Sullivan-Marx, E. M., Strumpf, N. E., Evans, L. K., Baumgarten, M., & Maislin, G. (1999). Predictors of continued physical restraint use in nursing home residents following restraint reduction efforts. *Journal of the American Geriatrics Society, 47,* 342–348.

Tetewsky, S. J., & Duffy, C. J. (1999). Visual loss and getting lost in Alzheimer's disease. *Neurology, 52,* 958–965.

Thomas, W. H. (1994). *The Eden Alternative: Nature, hope, & nursing homes.* Sherburne, NY: Eden Alternative Foundation.

Thomas, W. H. (1996). *Life worth living: How somebody you love can still enjoy life in a nursing home—The Eden Alternative.* Acton, MA: VanderWyk & Burnham.

Thomas, W. H. (1999). *The Eden Alternative Handbook: The art of building human habitats.* Sherburne, NY: Summer Hill Company.

Thomasma, D. C. (1995). Beyond autonomy to the person coping with illness. *Cambridge Quarterly of Healthcare Ethics, 4*(1), 12–22.

Tickle, E. H., & Hull, K. V. (1995). Family members' roles in long-term care. *MEDSURG Nursing, 4,* 300–304.

Tinetti, M. E., Liu, W.-L., Marottoli, R. A., & Ginter, S. F. (1991). Mechanical restraint use among residents of skilled nursing facilities: Prevalence, patterns, and predictors. *JAMA, 265*(4), 468–471.

Tolle, S. W., Rosenfeld, A. G., Tilden, V. P., & Park, Y. (1999). Oregon's low in-hospital death rates: What determines where people die and satisfaction with decisions on place of death? *Annals of Internal Medicine, 130,* 681–685.

Toulmin, S. (1981). The tyranny of principles. *Hastings Center Report, 11*(6), 31–39.

Travis, S. S., Loving, G., McClanahan, L., & Bernard, M. (2001). Hospitalization patterns and palliation in the last year of life among residents in long-term care. *The Gerontologist, 41,* 153–160.

Travis, S. S., Bernard, M., Dixon, S., McAuley, W. J., Loving, G., & McClanahan, L. (2002). Obstacles to palliation and end-of-life care in a long-term care facility. *The Gerontologist, 42,* 342–349.

Tune, L. E. (2001). Risperidone for the treatment of behavioral and psychological symptoms of dementia. *Journal of Clinical Psychiatry, 62*(suppl. 21), 29–32.

United States General Accounting Office (1998). *Alzheimer's disease: Estimates of prevalence in the United States.* Washington, DC: Author.

Vesperi, M. D. (1983). The reluctant consumer: Nursing home residents in the post Bergman era. In J. Sokolovsky (Ed.), *Growing old in different societies: Cross-cultural perspectives* (pp. 225–237). Belmont, CA: Wadsworth.

Vesperi, M. D. (1995). Nursing home research comes of age: Toward an ethnological perspective on long term care. In J. N. Henderson & M. D. Vesperi (Eds.), *The culture of long term care: Nursing home ethnography* (pp. 7–21). Westport, CT: Bergin & Garvey.

Vogelpohl, T. S., Beck, C. K., Heacock, P., & Mercer, S. O. (1996). "I can do it!" Dressing: Promoting independence through individualized strategies. *Journal of Gerontological Nursing, 22*(3), 39–42.

Volicer, L., & Bloom-Charette, L. (Eds.). (1999). *Enhancing the quality of life in advanced dementia.* Philadelphia: Taylor & Francis.

Vollen, K. H. (1996). Coping with difficult resident behaviors takes time. *Journal of Gerontological Nursing, 22*(8), 22–26.

Walker, M. U. (1993). Keeping moral space open. *Hastings Center Report, 23*(2), 33–40.

Watson, W., & Maxwell, R. (1977). *Human aging and dying: A study in sociocultural gerontology.* New York: St. Martin's Press.

Waymack, M. (2001). The ethical importance of home care. In M. B. Holstein & P. B. Mitzen (Eds.), *Ethics in community-based elder care* (pp. 51–59). New York: Springer.

Weaverdyck, S. E., Wittle, A., & deLaski-Smith, D. (1998). In-place progression: Lessons learned from the Huron Woods' staff. *Journal of Gerontological Nursing, 24*(1), 31–39.

Werhane, P. H., & Rorty, M. V. (2000). Organization ethics in healthcare. *Cambridge Quarterly of Healthcare Ethics, 9*(2), 145–146.

Wilson, S. A., & Daley, B. J. (1999). Family perspectives on dying in long-term care settings. *Journal of Gerontological Nursing, 25*(11), 19–25.

Wilson, S. A., Kovach, C. R., & Stearns, S. A. (1996). Hospice concepts in the care for end-stage dementia. *Geriatric Nursing, 17*(1), 6–10.

Williams, C. C. (1989). Liberation: Alternative to physical restraints. *The Gerontologist, 29*, 585–586.

Williams, C. C., & Finch, C. E. (1997). Physical restraint: Not fit for woman, man, or beast. *Journal of the American Geriatrics Society, 45*, 773–775.

Zerwekh, J. V. (1997). Do dying patients really need IV fluids? *American Journal of Nursing, 97*(3), 26–31.

Zilberfein, F. (1999). Coping with death: Anticipatory grief and bereavement. *Generations, 23*(1), 69–74.

Index

Activities, daily life and personal care, 3, 5, 10, 18–19, 39, 51, 57, 67–68, 85, 129, 137, 139, 152, 175. *See also* Bathing, Dressing, Eating, Grooming, Hair washing, Individualized/alternate care approaches, Oral hygiene, *and* Toileting

Activities, social and recreational opportunities and/or programming, 21, 30–31, 42–45, 48, 51–52, 57, 87–90, 98, 101–103, 105–106, 110, 117, 120, 125–126, 129, 140–145, 146, 168, 172, 176

Accusations/blaming, by person with dementia, 16, 35, 103, 107, 119. *See also* Paranoia *and* Suspiciousness

Advance directives, 13–14, 78–81, 92, 94, 98, 151–156, 174, 183, 188, 193–194; state-specific forms from Partnership for Caring, 14. *See also* Health care proxy/surrogate

Agitation/agitated behaviors, 5, 36, 41, 51, 77–78, 119–121, 123, 129, 157, 164, 166

Aggressive behaviors, 55, 76, 78, 116, 120–121, 137, 157. *See also* Combativeness

Aging in place, 31, 33–34, 56, 145–151, 176. *See also* Intra-institutional transfers

Agnosia, 8

AIDS or HIV-associated dementia (or AIDS dementia complex), 9

Alzheimer's disease: as a cause of dementia, 9; prevalence of, 1

Alzheimer's Disease and Related Disorders Association (ADRDA), 1–2, 12, 16, 23, 27–28, 196

Alzheimer's Disease Education and Referral Center (ADEAR), 28, 196

American Society for Bioethics and Humanities (ASBH), 186, 196

Anger/angry behavior, 4, 16, 17, 24, 68, 77, 109, 136, 140, 146, 157–158, 161

Aphasia, 8, 77. *See also* Communication *and* Language difficulties

Applied ethics. *See* Ethics.

Apraxia, 8, 78

Assisted living. *See* Community-based alternative living facilities

Autonomy/freedom of choice or to do as one wishes, 21, 44, 47, 53, 57, 63, 65, 74, 79, 92, 93, 96, 98, 116–117, 122, 125–126, 129, 138, 154, 160, 167, 176, 179. *See also* Resident preferences, wishes and choices *and* Residents' rights.

Bathing, 15, 19, 24, 39, 51, 67–68, 76, 78, 87, 135–140, 158

Belligerence, 22, 23, 110, 125

Beneficence/doing good, 63, 93, 96, 98, 105, 112, 122, 126, 132, 138, 143, 148, 154, 160, 167

Bioethics. *See* Ethics

![Springer / Publishing Company]
SPRINGER / PUBLISHING COMPANY

Applied Ethics in Nursing

Vicki Lachman, PhD, MBE, APRN, Editor

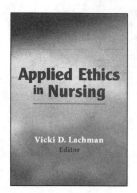

What constitutes informed consent?

What can I do if the patient lacks the capacity to make decisions?

How should I respond to a patient who requests my help in dying?

What is the rationale for giving a patient medication (chemical restraints) against his or her will?

What exactly are patient's rights and how do you advocate for your patients?

Applied Ethics in Nursing provides an easily understandable guide to the kind of ethical dilemmas you face in practice. Using a question-and-answer format along with numerous case studies, this text offers best practices and strategies for approaching the difficult problems commonly found in clinical practice.

This book also addresses organizational and institutional issues that can confound or promote ethically sound decision making. Each chapter ends with a resource list of websites and recommendations for further reading. The American Nurses' Association Code of Ethics for Nurses is used as a guide throughout, along with standards and guidelines from other major healthcare and governmental organizations.

Partial Contents

Part I: The Essence of Ethics and Advocacy in Nursing

Part II: Ethical Issues at the Beginning of Life

Part III: Ethical Issues with Vulnerable Populations

Part IV: The Right to Live and the Right to Die

Part V: Developing an Organizational Culture that Supports Ethical Behavior

Part VI: The Mix of Religion and Culture with Ethics

2005 · 216pp · 0-8261-7984-3 · softcover

11 West 42nd Street, New York, NY 10036-8002 • Fax: 212-941-7842
Order Toll-Free: 877-687-7476 • Order On-line: www.springerpub.com

SPRINGER PUBLISHING COMPANY

Bathing Without a Battle
Personal Care of Individuals with Dementia

Ann Louise Barrick, PhD
Joanne Rader, MN, RN, FAAN
Beverly Hoeffer, DNSc, RN, FAAN
Philip D. Sloane, MD, MPH, Editors

This book presents an individualized, problem solving approach to bathing and personal care of individuals with dementia. Based on extensive original research and clinical experience, the authors have developed strategies and techniques that work in both the institution and home settings. Their approach is also appropriate for caregiving activities other than bathing. Illustrations, charts, checklists, and relevant web sites are provided throughout.

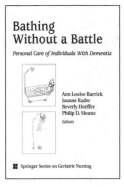

Bathing
Without a Battle
Personal Care of Individuals With Dementia

Ann Louise Barrick
Joanne Rader
Beverly Hoeffer
Philip D. Sloane
Editors

Springer Series on Geriatric Nursing

Partial Contents:

Part I: The Basics
Understanding the Battle • General Guidelines for Bathing Persons with Dementia • Assessing Behaviors • Selecting Individualized Solutions that Work

Part II: Special Concerns
Preserving Abilities: Finding the Best Level of Assistance • Managing Pain • Care of the Skin • Transfer Techniques • The Physical Environment of the Bathing Room • Equipment and Supplies

Part III: Supporting Caregiving Activities
Organizing Care Within the Institution or Home • Training Staff in Ways to Keep People Clean • Taking Care of Yourself: Strategies for Caregivers

2002 · 176pp · 0-8261-1507-1 · softcover

11 West 42nd Street, New York, NY 10036-8002 • Fax: 212-941-7842
Order Toll-Free: 877-687-7476 • Order On-line: www.springerpub.com

Geriatric Nursing

Growth of a Specialty

Priscilla Ebersole, RN PhD, FAAN
Terri Touhy, ND, APRN, BC

Learn the history of the development of geriatric nursing as a specialty, as well as the current state of geriatric nursing, from the stories of pioneers in this field. Through the history of those who laid the foundations for the profession, to the geriatric nurse leaders who continue the specialty today, see first-hand how geriatric nursing began, evolved, and continues to flourish.

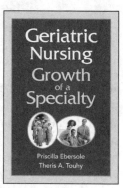

Covering the scope of the specialty:

• How to become a geriatric nurse
• Geriatric nursing organizations and publications
• Standards of practice
• Certification and licensure
• Future directions

This text provides both inspirational stories of nursing and practical information on how you can find resources, develop ideas, and access research in order to become a successful geriatric nurse.

Partial Contents

History and Development of Geriatric Nursing • Geriatric Nurse Pioneers and Their Contributions • Nurses in Action: The Second Generation • Geriatric Nurse Leaders Today • Recognition of Geriatric Care as a Specialty Practice • Geriatric Nursing Organizations and Affiliates • Educational Programs and Publications for Geriatric and Gerontological Nurses • Nursing Research and Geriatric Care • Elements of Attracting Nurses to the Field • Nursing and the Future Care of the Aged: Possibilities and Opportunities

2006 · 304pp · 0-8261-2649-9 · softcover

11 West 42nd Street, New York, NY 10036-8002 • Fax: 212-941-7842
Order Toll-Free: 877-687-7476 • Order On-line: www.springerpub.com